Making a
Psychopath

Making a Psychopath

My Journey into
7 Dangerous Minds

Dr Mark Freestone

EBURY
PRESS

1

Ebury Press, an imprint of Ebury Publishing
20 Vauxhall Bridge Road
London SW1V 2SA

Ebury Press is part of the Penguin Random House group of companies
whose addresses can be found at global.penguinrandomhouse.com

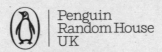

First published by Ebury Press in 2020

www.penguin.co.uk

A CIP catalogue record for this book is available from
the British Library

ISBN 9781529106541

Typeset in 11.5/18.5 pt New Century Schoolbook LT Std
by Integra Software Services Pvt. Ltd, Pondicherry

Printed and bound in Great Britain by Clays Ltd, Elcograf S.p.A.

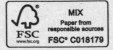

Penguin Random House is committed to a
sustainable future for our business, our readers
and our planet. This book is made from Forest
Stewardship Council® certified paper.

Of course, this book is for Lotte,
Edward and Albert.

Contents

Preface

'We want your help with a character: it's a TV show about a female assassin. Who's also a psychopath.'

My face rested slowly into the palm of my hand. Fortunately for everyone, this wasn't visible to the very lovely and well-meaning person on the phone.

'Umm ...' I stalled, trying not to sigh too audibly. Everyone knows (don't they?) that women are rarely psychopaths and almost never assassins. Apart from anything else, male assassins have the 'killing game' tied down hard and tend to give horrible new meanings to the phrase 'rampant misogyny'.

Wait, though: there was Ulrike Meinhof, right? Brigitte Mohnhaupt? Aileen Wuornos? They were women, and they killed a lot of people – for political reasons at least. Sort of. Maybe I could work with this: a misunderstood, isolated weirdo who is recruited into a strange sect on the fringes of society.

'We also want her to be really glamorous and sexy.'

I made a funny noise like someone who had spent two years studying for an A-level English paper on Shakespeare only to turn over their exam and find questions about Emily Dickinson. I had to make this wish-list into a real, credible psychopath. Why did I ever get involved in working with TV anyway?

The beginning of this story reaches back to the early 2000s, when I – clutching my just-printed Sociology PhD – secured some research funding to do an investigation study of the Dangerous and Severe Personality Disorder (DSPD) Programme in England and Wales. DSPD was supposed to be a shining new hope of treatment for people with severe personality disorders, especially antisocial personality disorder (sociopathy) and psychopathy. There was a huge sense of therapeutic optimism back then, and a dose of apparently healthy arrogance: no other country in the world had managed to reliably treat psychopaths before, but that was only because the British hadn't tried it on this kind of scale.[1]

Ignoring several pointed statements of concern from highly experienced psychiatrists and psychologists, between 2002 and 2005 four new special high-security units in prisons and hospitals in the UK were opened to some of Britain's most dangerous and uncontainable men and women … and me. Between 2004 and 2013 I worked in and around these new units, talking to hundreds of prisoners and staff and trying to understand what this system was and how it was going to make a difference where nothing else had. Being neither a forensic psychologist nor a psychiatrist, I had no real concept of what a psychopath was when I began, and I had to learn from the ground up what made these prisoners different.

Over these years I gained a huge amount of experience with men diagnosed with psychopathy, and with the brave people who volunteered to work with them through the DSPD Programme and beyond. Some of the work was formal, meeting with patients and prisoners to conduct assessment or treatment under the supervision of a psychologist or psychiatrist, or my own research; and some of it was informal, meeting patients and staff on the ward and talking about whatever was on the wind, playing chess or guitar with inmates.

It was being contacted to work on *Killing Eve*, and drawing on my experiences with psychopaths, some of which made their way into the television series in one form or another to help the writers shape the story and characters, that made me think about these experiences again. Villanelle is such a curiously compelling character. Both in the series and Luke Jennings' original *Villanelle* novellas, she is a terrible, terrible person: devoid of warmth, empathy, relationship skills, humility or genuine emotion, who not only kills people for money but also because she thinks it's funny, or simply because it's more convenient than having to tolerate relationships with them. Yet, something about her draws people in: perhaps people identify with parts of her character, or perhaps they envy the chaos she brings with her.

Of course, Villanelle is fiction. And although we tried to make her as real as possible, I realised that my own stories could give a window into what it's like interacting with people with a diagnosis of psychopathy, and that they could also show that psychopaths are not all one and the same. Although it does seem that criminal psychopaths have no problem acting out in detail some of the darkest things that would make most of us feel guilty if we only dreamed them, one of the few things about psychopaths I'm absolutely sure of is that psychopathy in itself is not a *reason* or a *cause* for doing anything.

I hope this book gives people whose interest, of whatever kind, was piqued by Villanelle and characters like her a chance to understand a bit more about the very misunderstood disorder – or more likely disorders – we call psychopathy. Taking a chapter each for seven types of patient, I am going to show how very diverse criminal psychopaths are in their backgrounds, their characters and their ways of being dangerous. From the horrifically violent gang leader to the man who always ends up hurting those who help him, what the people in this book all have in common is that they have done at least one terrible thing to another person and they can't quite understand why the rest of society is making such a fuss about it.

Introduction

Does the world need another book on psychopaths?[1] After all, it seems we have heard or read just about everything there is to say about this most misunderstood of characters. Are they evil from birth? Are they created by perverse or abusive family dynamics? Why do some psychopaths make for such compelling fictional characters? Is my ex or boss a psychopath?

I am not a psychiatrist, someone who diagnoses and treats mental disorders, nor a forensic psychologist, who studies the minds, brains and behaviour of criminals, although I have worked extensively with some of the most influential and experienced members of both professions. My background is a bit different: I originally trained in sociology, a discipline mainly concerned with understanding patterns of relationships and social interaction and which rarely deals with the individual. However, I have worked directly with criminal psychopaths in secure hospitals and in the community for over 15 years. I have eaten with psychopaths, laughed and cried with them. I have seen them bleed and, in one case, die. They have manipulated me; I have probably manipulated them. And many words have been said – usually not by me – that should never be said by one human to another.

Throughout this time, conducting research, performing assessments and running treatment groups, I have built up both a wealth of experience of how psychopaths interact with people, and a resolute scepticism about the way that psychiatry and forensic psychology views psychopaths. Today I work in a psychiatry department that prides itself on a bio-psychosocial understanding of mental disorder, which means that we always try to understand the influence of the circumstances in which people grew up on their adult lives, when thinking about mental disorder. This is critically important in formulating a treatment plan that can help to persuade that person that there are positive reasons to change, and to avoid recreating the traumatic, abusive or neglectful environments of their childhood.

My belief is that to understand people we should always focus on relationships rather than traits and diagnosis, and so I feel I can offer a slightly different perspective on this most misunderstood of personalities. Psychopaths don't exist in a vacuum: their disorder is about the way they understand and interact with other people; about the relationships they form. One of the questions I sometimes ask my students is whether a psychopath would be able to survive on a desert island far away from other humans. My answer to this is: yes, absolutely. Someone with a diagnosis of, say, schizophrenia or dementia would be unlikely to cope in such an isolated setting on their own and would probably perish. I think a psychopath would thrive.

I also hope I can offer some clarity about what makes a psychopath and whether they can change. There are too many contradictory statements about what the term 'psychopath' means and whether treatment always makes psychopaths worse rather than better. There's a smorgasbord of stubborn misconceptions about people with a psychopathic disorder that come partly from our tendency – and this was certainly the perspective I had when I first started working in secure mental health services in 2004 – to think of psychopathy as a footnote for a kind of supervillain, bereft of a moral compass and totally Machiavellian in their expert manipulation of others. In fact, years of experience have taught me that the reality is less dramatic, but perhaps far more unsettling: that psychopaths are, in the vast majority, not experts in much at all, and certainly not intellectual puppet masters like Thomas Harris's Hannibal Lecter. Rather, they are individuals who, through a toxic and statistically unlikely combination of genetic bad luck and a desperate emotionally, physically or financially deprived upbringing, have come to lack some of the most basic social skills, powers of reasoning and emotional responses that contribute so much to making us human. This, I aim to show, is what makes a psychopath.

I want to show how a single word, 'psychopath', is far too narrow a term to capture the diversity of people who have attracted the label. I want to highlight the kind of disturbed environments that create psychopaths and the 'containers' – prison and, to a lesser extent, psychiatric hospitals – that perpetuate their social and personal dysfunction, allowing them to hone their skills of manipulation and sadism.

My hope is that the anonymised case studies in this book, each one an amalgamation of the characters who I have come across in my professional life, help to humanise psychopaths, and help the reader understand why it is so difficult for these men and women to form the kinds of social and emotional relationships we take for granted.

I am interested in whether it is fair to morally judge psychopaths and whether there is a degree of complicity between all of us, professionals and the general public alike, in consigning them to the dustbin of humanity. I think that, more often, professionals working in mental health and criminal justice systems adopt the easier and attractive judgemental perspective on psychopaths, perceiving them as 'impossible to rehabilitate' or 'naturally evil'. This way, when things go wrong and someone loses their job for a breach of professional ethics for allowing themselves to be manipulated by a psychopath, we comfort ourselves with the notion that the psychopath is simply a genetic aberration we cannot help but can only be intimidated or controlled by. Similarly, if clinicians have nothing to offer someone with psychopathy, this becomes a self-fulfilling prophecy: 'I can't help you, so you must be bad'.[2]

Combine this with the psychopath's tendency towards violence, manipulation and controlling behaviour, and you'll find that working with them is very rarely a straightforward or satisfying task.

Psychopaths tend to reoffend more prolifically and more quickly than other offenders: one study says that up to 90 per cent of psychopathic offenders will be reconvicted of a violent offence within 20 years.[3] Diligence and persistence are often rewarded with disappointment and frustration, and sometimes a complaint or a colourful metaphor about your parentage.

This book describes composites of people I have dealt with in my career and some publicly visible ones. They include Danny, a man who is more of a danger to himself than to anyone else. Eddie, who has a terrifying history of violence but has turned away from that life and found empathy and remorse. And Angela, a woman who perhaps scares me more than any of the men I describe. In some way each story challenges the misconceptions about psychopaths, and they will hopefully give you a different perspective on the disorder and the kind of person that springs to mind when we use the word.

Chapter One
The Masks of Psychopathy

Although psychopathy has been one of the most important and written-about topics of forensic psychiatry and psychology over the last 30 years, it's astonishing how little we really understand it. In part, this makes sense: psychopaths are not common, the largest group of them are in the criminal justice system, and increasingly doing research in prisons and forensic hospitals is expensive, complex and often unrewarding. Not to mention, of course, that most psychopaths in prison are probably quite bored and, well, psychopathic: meaning that some of them will be entirely disinterested in engaging in research at all – after all, what would they gain? – and another group will see any research project as an opportunity to present themselves in a particular, usually favourable, light that doesn't have any basis in reality. Or they'll just tell some fantastic whoppers and watch the researcher squirm as they try to weight social convention against the urge to laugh, scream or slap their research participant (or all three). This is a bit of a shame, because in the early 2000s a lot of progress was made in trying to understand that there were probably several different kinds of psychopath, and that using a single word to describe them all was increasingly problematic.

I want to tease apart the idea that the word 'psychopath' or the diagnosis of 'psychopathy' refers to a single type of person, instantly recognisable from just about every television programme with a one-dimensional bad guy (or gal, more of which later): in fact, people with a diagnosis of psychopathy can differ quite fundamentally from each other in several significant ways. Understanding this and why it might be will prepare you a bit for the variety of presentations – the variety of 'masks' that psychopaths wear, or that we project on to them – that we'll meet in the chapters that follow.

Fifteen Thousand Paper Psychopaths

How can one diagnosis mean many things? Well, for a start, we might want to think about the Psychopathy Checklist, Revised (PCL-R)[1], the gold standard psychopathy assessment used by forensic psychologists and psychiatrists across the world, which consists of 20 items relating to distinctive traits of a psychopath, each rateable between 0 and 2. If we take the more conservative threshold used in the United States, someone needs a score of 30 on the PCL-R to be diagnosed as a 'clinical psychopath'. This means, as Jon Ronson points out in his terrific book on the subject of the PCL-R, *The Psychopath Test,* that there are 15,504 different combinations of items[2] that would result in someone meeting the threshold, each representing a different cluster of different traits: over 15,000 different ways to be a psychopath.

To make matters more complex, there are two very different constellations or factors within the PCL-R. One is a group of traits, or personality features, that relate to antisocial behaviour: impulsivity, poor behavioural controls, criminal convictions and so on. People with this group of traits tend to show antisocial behaviour during their early adult life: drug addiction, offending, bankruptcy, homelessness and a tendency towards making decisions without planning. At around the age of 30, however, their criminality and antisocial behaviour seem to 'burn out'[3] and they desist in most cases from this kind of criminal or self-destructive behaviour. The second group usually has this antisocial tendency too, but also a further set of personality traits – such as callousness, shallow emotions and a lack of remorse for their acts – that tend to be more durable over time and which are genetically based.[4] These traits never really change throughout a lifespan,[5] meaning that people with this group won't ever fully find a way of empathising with others or understanding emotions. This also means that, without treatment, they will never be truly 'safe' within society.

One of the biggest questions facing psychopathy research is whether psychopaths are also necessarily criminals. Hervey Cleckley was the first psychiatrist to write about psychopaths in detail, and his book *The Mask of Sanity*,[6] published in 1941, didn't specify anything about criminality or violence in his description of the disorder. In fact, his understanding of psychopaths was very different to ours today. Rather than cool, calculating criminals, Cleckley believed that psychopaths were 'morally insane'; that they were unable to tell right from wrong and therefore just as 'mad' as people with a psychotic illness like schizophrenia, albeit their madness affected a different part of the brain relating to moral reasoning, not perception. However, he suggested that in a psychopath madness was 'concealed' by a mask of social awareness that hid the madness, effectively tricking those around them into thinking they were sane. It was their inability to learn from mistakes, to feel remorse for those they hurt or to empathise with emotions in others that revealed the deep inner disturbance, marking them out as psychopaths.

Despite acknowledging lack of remorse as a core aspect of psychopathy, Cleckley did not make any association between psychopathy and crime; that only came later with Robert Hare's Psychopathy

Checklist[7] in 1980. This was based on Cleckley's work but had several advantages: rather than a theoretical description of a concept, Hare gave a set of clear and measurable criteria, in the form of a checklist, which measured how psychopathic someone was on a scale. Anyone who has worked in applied psychology knows how important this is. Once a concept is 'testable' it is useable in clinical practice, and – in the case of a measure that relates to crime as well as mental disorder – forensic and criminal work, too.

It was with the second edition of the checklist, the PCL-R[8], that Hare did something that has divided understanding of psychopathy ever since: he incorporated both criminal and behavioural tendencies into his checklist. In many respects this was a great decision: it allowed the checklist to be used in courts, where it was not just an assessment of a clinical condition but, as a hybrid measure, could also perform a fair assessment of a convicted offender's chances of reoffending. However, it also leads to a fundamental change in the way we think about psychopaths, from people with a moral deficiency similar to madness, to people who are primarily criminals whose emotional and thinking deficits make them more suited to, and predisposed to, crime.

A Different Brain?

We now have a lot more research available to us about the causes of psychopathy, how it manifests in the brain, and in the genetic profile of people with the disorder, and we know it is not the case that all psychopaths are necessarily criminals. We'll look at the brain first.

The high quality brain-imaging equipment that became available in the early twenty-first century has shown that there are two very specific regions of psychopaths' brains that differ significantly from those of people without psychopathy, and that these brain regions are linked to specific kinds of emotional and cognitive processing that are deficient in psychopaths.

The first of these two regions is the prefrontal cortex, a region shaped like a half-moon that takes up most of the frontal lobe of your brain, just behind your brows. First-year psychology students almost all get a lecture on the case of Phineas Gage, the nineteenth-century Australian rail worker who took a tamping iron – a two-metre piece of iron used to 'pin down' rail tracks – through his eye socket and not only survived, but did so with most of his cognitive abilities intact. However, the iron significantly damaged Gage's prefrontal cortex[9] and as a result his personality was completely altered: he become irritable and prone to aggressive mood swings, although he could still function tolerably in society; enough to hold down a job after his recovery from the injury.[10]

Similarly, I have worked with patients who have a diagnosis of an 'organic' personality disorder: this means that the diagnosing doctor(s) believe that they have isolated the cause of the psychopathy or sociopathy to a specific, neurological cause. One patient I worked with had had a very difficult birth where there was damage to their frontal lobe owing to obstetric forceps. (This is a vanishingly rare thing to happen: only around five in a thousand births in the UK will result in brain injury, and the majority of these will be due to oxygen deprivation to the baby's brain,[11] not a direct physical injury.) My patient had terribly dysregulated behaviour: they spoke normally and showed good intellectual development (played a mean game of chess), but almost seemed incapable of making rational decisions or sticking to them without being overcome with nearly hysterical levels of emotion: rage, despair, elation, contempt, guilt, anger, sadness, all within minutes of each other.

This is because the prefrontal cortex and its near neighbour, the orbitofrontal cortex ('orbit' being the area around the eye), govern our ability to make good decisions based on available information, and in particular our expectation of how society will respond to us when we fail to conform to social rules and norms, for example by breaking the law. [12] In a psychopath, these areas, absent or severely damaged in Phineas Gage, show significantly lower activation;[13] that is, the neurons in that part of the brain light up less than usual in a brain-imaging machine, indicating less activity, and appear to be linked to an inability to learn from experience.

The second region that is different in psychopaths is the amygdala, a small area in the very centre of the brain, right at the top of the brain stem, in what we know as the 'limbic' system. The amygdala is closely linked to a lot of brain regions and we think it plays a key, critical role in our ability to process and understand emotion. I say 'we think' because this is a part of the brain that is deep in the grey matter at the base of the skull and we have no lucky anecdotal evidence, such as the case of Phineas Gage, to help us determine its exact purpose.

Any injury that penetrated to the amygdala would almost certainly result in death because of the importance of the surrounding brain tissue to essential things like breathing and keeping your heart beating. Instead, all we have to go on are observational studies that show a link between people with reduced activation – which is a pretty general idea as we don't know how much activation is 'normal' – and problems in recognising emotions, particularly fear, disgust or sadness, in faces.[14] Clearly, someone who is unable to recognise emotion would have difficulties in expressing remorse or empathy with others because they would not even see why these responses would be necessary; and there we have the 'void' at the core of the psychopath.

Touching the Void

Putting this together, we have pretty good, although not definitive, evidence that psychopaths have something different about their brain make-up that probably means they are unable to make calculations about risk, or to recognise and respond to emotions in others. However, even people with quite severe brain abnormalities in these areas can lead perfectly healthy, normal lives, and this brings me to a second fascinating case: that of James H. Fallon, a well-known American neuropsychologist.

James (Jim) Fallon is a family man with a very successful career in neuropsychology. I strongly recommend his excellent, fascinating and unsettling account of his own experiences *The Psychopath Inside*[15] and his compelling TED talk. To cut a long story short, however, Jim was conducting some standard research using PET scans (a kind of early magnetic resonance imagining or MRI technique) when he noticed that one of the scans showed exceptionally low activity in areas of the amygdala, prefrontal cortex and limbic system. 'Huh, this guy is a regular psychopathic murderer,' he flippantly thought, only to realise that the scan was actually from a supposedly 'healthy' control. When he checked the patient ID he further noticed that the healthy control was listed as a 'Dr J. Fallon': the neuroscientist himself was a psychopath. He then sought out his genealogical records and realised that he had several ancestors who had been killers, and quite possibly psychopaths. Next, he tested his DNA profile, which revealed he had the 'warrior' version of the MAO-A gene, an unusual genetic profile typically found in people who have committed a few murders.

Jim's family had always been aware that he was emotionally distant, paid little or no attention to social niceties and was known for a bit of a temper. But he was also a pretty big deal in academic circles before this took place. He had built his scientific career on well-conducted neuroscience, which is, well ... hard. You can't 'blag' your way as a neuroscientist (believe me, I've tried): it requires a technical understanding of both physiology and complicated research techniques, an eye for detail, an ability to think in the abstract and very high levels of patience. None of these things are typically associated with psychopaths, nor any of the patients and prisoners I have worked with. Jim was such a big deal, in fact, that the knowledge that he had all the genetic and physiological traits of a psychopath didn't really hurt his career, except to hook him up with a book deal and a lot of media attention. He explained in one interview: 'I know something's wrong [with me]; I just don't care ... I don't give a shit.'

So here we have the first mask of psychopathy: not all psychopaths are the same, and some are unrecognisable from each other. Jim's case highlights some very serious questions about the nature of criminal psychopathy and where it comes from, and why despite all the genetics and the brain structure he would never make the grade on the Psychopath Test. Yes, brain structure and genes play a part, but experience has taught me that there are some clear regularities about the past of the people I have worked with. I say this because I have never, ever met a psychopathic criminal, much less a killer, who magically sprang from a near-perfect background. Some psychopaths come from relatively (or even very) privileged homes, or families where on the surface all can seem well; however, scratch beneath that surface and there is always something amiss. This can manifest in obvious ways – perhaps a parent with a drink problem, or a violent relationship between the mother and father – or it can be more subtle – a disproportionate allocation of love for one child at the expense of another, or a paternal figure who believes in discipline at the expense of any human connection. These disruptions target the vital bond or 'attachment'[16] between parents and their children, meaning that the children lack a clear sense of who they should be or how they should behave. It seems that when a child's sense of identity and security is absent or distorted in this way, this is fertile ground for the development of a criminal psychopath as the child's genes, their character, interacts with their environment.

Someone recently challenged me on this theory, citing the American serial killer Ted Bundy as someone who was widely believed to be a psychopath[17] but had a 'normal' upbringing. However, reading closely between the lines, Bundy's early life shows a pattern of highly distorted role models and relationships: confusion about the true identity of his father – never a stable basis for a young man to develop a secure sense of self – and a grandiose, patriarchal grandfather[18] who provided exactly the kind of callous, remorseless and aggressive role model that any budding psychopath needs. The great psychoanalyst Phyllis Greenacre, one of the first people to write about psychopaths, noted as long ago as 1945, before Bundy and long before *The Psychopath Test*, how many psychopaths seemed to come from families where the father was 'an unusually prominent or respected man'.[19]

Now, absolutely, some people have suffered through terrible upbringings far worse than this, sometimes with terrifying parental figures, and yet turned into decent, respectable members of society. I am good friends with someone who has suffered terrible sexual and emotional abuse at the hands of their father and brother, yet they have a life, a partner, two children and their own business, all of whom they are absolutely dedicated to. They wear the marks of their traumatic childhood almost like battle scars: they have an endearingly pragmatic and resolute internal formulation that these awful experiences have made them who they are today, and that was someone to be proud of, not feel guilty about. This friend told me once that because of their own childhood they recognised the value of love and family, and that they would never endanger either now they are an adult with their own children.

Here is the second mask of psychopathy: whether someone will be a psychopath or not does not depend only on their upbringing but on a complex interplay between early experience and genetics, both of which play a part in the formation of the adult brain. Two particular genetic patterns stand out: firstly, the particular type MAO-A gene that affected Jim Fallon; and secondly a particular phenotype – that is, an expression of particular genetic patterns – called 'callous unemotional traits' that are first noticed in children.

'Callous unemotionality' is a trait in the Psychopathy Checklist, but it's quite rare for it to be applied to children; however, it is children aged 12 or younger who start to show callous unemotional traits – that is, a disregard for the impact of their actions on other people and a general lack of emotional range or recognition – who tend to have the worst outcomes for criminality and adult psychopathy. This tendency is different to those children who don't show callous unemotionality until young adulthood (i.e. as teenagers) and has been shown by studies of twins to be unaffected by social class, education or parenting.[20] This doesn't mean that Lionel Shriver's book *We Need to Talk about Kevin*, where a young boy seems to spring from the womb as a ready-made psychopath, is intended as a cautionary tale to any would-be parents. Not all children with callous unemotional traits develop into an adult psychopath and not all adult psychopaths had these traits as children (or at least, as far as we know). Rather, I think it's the book's ambiguity about whether the mother is an honest narrator about her relationship with her son that is the fundamental conceit: are the parents truly blameless victims of their psychopathic offspring, or have they somehow brought this fate upon themselves? In my experience, and to summarise the findings from research, the answer to this question is almost certainly 'the latter': the way parents act towards their children has huge implications for the development of psychopathy.

Killer Women: Psychopaths or Unicorns?

The third and final mask of psychopathy is the way it manifests through gender. A key part of what I think makes *Killing Eve* an effective thriller, and something that took a lot of time and discussion to get right in the early writing meetings, was whether the psychopathic assassin Villanelle could be made out to be a 'true' – in the sense of clinically accurate – psychopath. Why was this so challenging? Because 'true' female psychopaths are a highly elusive breed. Firstly, there are very, very few of them: when the UK government first commissioned secure prison and hospital places for dangerous people with severe personality disorders for the DSPD Programme, they estimated that the population of men they were serving was around 2,000. However, the highest estimate they could come up for women dangerous and psychopathic enough to warrant specialised care for their personality disorder was only 40, or 1 female psychopath for every 50 males. If we accept the (generous) estimate that there are about 3 psychopaths in every 1,000 men, this means that only 6 in every 100,000 women will be diagnosable as a psychopath using the PCL-R checklist, making about 200 female psychopaths in the UK. In other words, they are very rare, if we accept that the PCL-R is a good way of assessing women for psychopathy.

However, current understandings suggest that female psychopaths don't present or behave in the same way as male psychopaths. Scottish forensic psychologist Caroline Logan has written some of the most interesting work on this difference, and in a recent article she summarised our cultural conceptions of the female psychopath as a 'femme fatale':[21] not someone who was necessarily physically harmful towards others – although we will look at Angela Simpson, an interesting case that challenges this misconception, later on – but rather who harms and damages relationships and well-being psychologically. Logan talks about how male psychopaths tend to focus their energies on control, or the mastery of their environment and others around them, where female psychopaths are much more focused on the manipulation of relationships. She uses the example of the character of the Marquise de Merteuil in *Les Liaisons Dangereuses* (or Kathryn Merteuil in the 1999 film *Cruel Intentions*) who seeks to carry out revenge by playing characters' desires off against one another to her own benefit. Like a male psychopath, she does this through deceit and lies, without any expression of empathy or remorse, and in apparently full knowledge of the damage her actions will do.

There are dozens of other expressions of this kind of arch female manipulator in fiction: from Hedda Gabler in Ibsen's play of the same name (1896), to Sula Peace in Toni Morrison's *Sula* (1973) and more recently in Tana French's *In the Woods* (2007). Often in these stories there is violence done, but it is rarely, if ever, by the female antagonist: rather, other characters – frequently men – are manipulated into hurting themselves or others with threats or promises.

It's all very well to learn from fiction, but what do we know about female psychopaths in real life? The answer is that research is patchy, probably because there are so few women who meet these criteria. The first observation to make is that yes, there are a small number of women – the 40 or so we discussed earlier – who would score highly enough on the PCL-R to qualify as criminal psychopaths. The second, more complex idea is: it is very possible that women with psychopathy often have very different psychological and criminal profiles to men. Some of the items in the PCL-R might have very different interpretations when applied to women rather than men: for example, the item relating to a 'parasitic lifestyle' would be clearly applied to a man who was financially dependent on a woman, but cultural considerations might well mean that a woman being financially dependent upon a man is not convincing evidence of psychopathy.[22] Similarly, 'promiscuous sexual behaviour', another PCL-R item, might have different underlying motivations and meanings between men and women: for men this behaviour might be about status and sensation-seeking, whereas for women it might be more related to power and manipulation.[23] So, qualifying the previous answer of yes, the maybe response cautions us that even women who score highly on the PCL-R may not have the same motivations for their behaviour or psychological profile as men.

The third point is that there are probably no 'real' female psychopaths who resemble Villanelle's psychopathic assassin in *Killing Eve*. If we mean by that that they use personal violence as well as psychological intimidation and sexual manipulation to achieve their goals, and show no remorse for their violent actions, then the answer is there are no real precedents for this. In fact, there is even some contradictory evidence: a Dutch study found that highly psychopathic women were actually *less* likely to commit homicide than men,[24] which lends some support to the idea that female psychopaths eschew violence in favour of relationship-based manipulation. There are exceptions: Angela Simpson, who we'll discuss in chapter seven, who presents with a very 'male' form of psychopathy; and Aileen Wuornos, who murdered six men in the United States in the late 1980s and who was found to have a very high PCL-R score of 32 out of 40.[25] However, up until her execution in 2002 she gave very different and inconsistent accounts of her offending and her feelings of remorse (or otherwise) towards her victims; she was also diagnosed with borderline personality disorder, which is a condition almost incompatible with psychopathy, with symptoms including extreme emotional dysregulation and an unstable self-identity. There is also a plausible narrative for a lot of the killings beyond simple gratification or violence for violence's sake: Wuornos repeatedly stated that the killings were self-defence as she believed the victims were planning to rape her. Whether they were or not, if she perceived this level of threat it would constitute a degree of motivation that would not require someone to be psychopathic in order to act.

Moving Things Forward

What can all these people have in common: a blue-collar worker who becomes sociopathic after a brain injury, a New York professor who is well socially integrated but struggles to relate to other people, a group of kids who start from an early age to show signs of an uncaring attitude towards their peers and a female psychopath who might not be a psychopath at all? It's not an easy question to answer, but it's not one we can ignore: psychopathy is again and again shown to be so strongly related to risk of violence,[26] social deviance including risky drug use and financial instability,[27] and poor likelihood of successful treatment, rehabilitation or 'recovery'. How is it possible to hit this moving target: to understand what a psychopath is, bring together the seemingly contradictory strands of research, and to try to do something constructive about improving the prospects of people with this most misunderstood disorder?

Psychopathy, as we best understand it, which is an uneasy alliance between a checklist of controlling and antisocial behaviours matched with a number of structural deficits in the brain, explains a fair bit about why some people are more likely to make a risky or interpersonally damaging choice in each situation. However, it doesn't often offer a convincing or satisfying motive for anything: someone with a diagnosis of schizophrenia may have a delusional belief that their friend is secretly plotting to murder them and hear a voice telling them to poison their tea, but psychopathy offers no such clear causal pathways from someone's internal world to their behaviours.

One of the best examples I can think of is one I still go over with my students today: a man I will call Ben, a life-sentenced prisoner. Ben was sent to prison for armed robbery after a failed attack on an armoured money van, which had been coordinated by his stepfather. When Ben was released from prison, he was fixated on taking revenge for what he saw as a 'set-up', where his stepfather had led to him being sent to prison. After just two weeks on release he put together a 'tool bag' of hammers, knives, rope and a saw, and set off with the very explicit intent of killing his stepfather. However, along the way he met an old friend who persuaded him to come to the pub for a drink. Over a few beers, Ben confessed what he was planning, and the friend persuaded him that it wasn't worth it: Ben had only just come out of a long prison sentence, why was he so keen to go back there? Ben saw sense, and the two of them stayed until closing time, then set off for home. The friend, engaging in what sounds like drunken banter, told Ben he was a 'pussy' for being talked out of his murderous plot so easily: so Ben grabbed the hammer from his bag, and beat his friend to death with it.

Now don't get me wrong: Ben was deeply psychopathic. He didn't 'get' remorse, was a career criminal (albeit a very bad one as he was always getting caught) and grandiose in his sense of entitlement to be violent to people who wronged him. He planned a very serious offence out of nothing but a misguided sense of revenge for a damaged ego: and on the way to carry this out, he impulsively decided not go to go through with it, until he received another blow to his ego that he responded to with sudden homicidal rage. Knowing Ben was a psychopath doesn't really explain this, though: rather, it's his specific personality, his extreme ego vulnerability and hair trigger that contributed to the murder that day. In other words, the actions of psychopaths still very much need an explanation beyond 'they are a psychopath'.

It is very, very easy to write bad fictional psychopathic characters: 'Ahmed was dangerous ... because he was a psychopath'; and it is very hard to

write good ones. This is because the 'void' at the centre of the psychopathic mind, the fleeting displays
of deep emotion (shallow affect) and cold-blooded
nature, isn't very interesting in itself. This 'void'
has to be overlaid onto a complex developmental
history and set of desires and motivations, as it
always is in real life. Hannibal Lecter's relationship with Clarice Starling is one example. What
does Lecter want from Clarice: a protégé? But she
is repulsed by his killing. A lover? He is homosex-
ual. A daughter? This is a psychopath, incapable of
attachment. The key, of course, is that this is never
made explicit and we are made to guess what Lecter thinks this relationship is.

Psychopathic disorder wears masks on many
levels. Psychopathy can hide in plain sight, and
our confusion about its core traits makes it very
difficult to make a clear determination about
whether someone is or isn't a psychopath, unless
they are a very 'typical' male criminal who had
serious behavioural problems as a child. How can
we take a concept seriously, though, if the difference between a psychopath and a non-psychopath

is simply whether they were or were not convicted of a crime? What bearing can the accurate (or inaccurate) functioning of the justice system possibly have on one person's psychological make-up? *American Psycho*'s Patrick Bateman shows that wealth and privilege can confound our understandings of culpability and personality, and how unfair that is in a world where so many people will have been sentenced to death because of a supposed diagnosis of psychopathic disorder.

The people I describe in the coming chapters are intended to help show that a 'psychopath' often has far more to them than a simple diagnosis. Like all of us, they are complex individuals with idiosyncratic motivations, beliefs, desires and criminal offences, not reducible to the fact that they are psychopaths. However, it is because they are psychopaths that we need to take notice of them: in every case these men and women have committed very serious crimes, some of them truly horrific, and there is every likelihood that they will do so again.

Chapter Two
Paul, The Hitman

Working in large institutions – prisons, hospitals, bail hostels – with people who have committed serious crimes is hard, draining work. The people you are working with are at once potentially dangerous, having committed at least one serious crime and being dissatisfied with their incarceration, and yet also highly vulnerable. This means that your job as a professional is incredibly difficult: you are working with people in a place they do not want to be, trying to give them a reason to change that they do not want and trying to avoid giving them the opportunity to do harm to you, which a number of them certainly do. On top of that, criminals with personality disorders such as psychopathy are hard to rehabilitate: there is no clear treatment for their mental disorder and they are often very keen to recreate the life they came from – usually one defined by drugs and violence – within the prison. This means that prisons themselves are hard places. Most of the older jails with any kind of interesting Victorian architecture are now long gone, victims of health and safety regulations that require plumbing for toilets rather than slop buckets and clear lines of sight around the wings so people cannot get up to nefarious deeds in the shadows. What is left are cold, concrete institutions that are often characterised by bare, whitewashed walls. Maximum-security prisons are perhaps the worst: the walls are higher and supplemented by extra-high wire fences and helicopter wire.

Nobody, in any institution I worked in, was as adroit at bringing their outside life with them into prison as Paul. I first met him in a high-security prison together with a group of other prisoners who were discussing their upcoming treatment with a psychologist. This was a new service, part of the DSPD service, established in a prison to work with serious offenders who had previously been considered 'untreatable' because of their psychopathy or other serious personality disorder. My job at the time was to observe meetings like these to try to understand and write about the kind of culture created when you tried to rehabilitate the apparently unrehabilitatable; how relationships were formed between staff and prisoners who might have been in solitary confinement for years or never had a parole meeting where they had a chance of being released from prison.

Most of the prisoners in the group looked anxious, probably rightly, as most of them had life sentences and realised that this might be their last chance to ever get out of prison. However, nobody had any idea about what 'treatment' was, beyond a couple of stitches from the nurse after a fight in the canteen. One man in the group held the prison's record for solitary confinement: he had been locked up on his own for six years, and now even sitting next to other people caused him to sweat profusely and look nervously at the blank wall behind him several times per minute. I imagined that after a solitary cell measuring eight by ten feet, even this

poky, windowless prison meeting room, which barely held eight chairs and a filing cabinet, must have
felt impossibly open and exposed. Another man, also
sweating, wore a pair of what I came to learn were
known as 'nonce glasses': glasses with photoreact-
ive lenses that darken in bright light to protect the
eyes, and to which sex offenders are inexplicably
yet compulsively drawn. I say inexplicably because
every other prisoner and staff member seems to
know that wearing them is pretty much a mem-
bership card to the 'nonce club' so nobody else ever
does – violent offenders looking to victimise a nonce
thus always know exactly where to start.

In the middle of this motley group, sitting in
a slump that made him practically horizontal,
manspreading like it was going out of fashion,
was when I first laid eyes on Paul. His mouth was
twisted in the odd, mirthless expression of someone who feels nothing but contempt for anything
around him but feels he should probably disguise
that fact in his best interests.

'I wonder what everyone's expectations are of
today?' asked the female psychologist, following

an approved line of Socratic questioning and doing everyone the courtesy of looking genuinely interested in the answers.

'Get the fuck out of this place,' quipped Paul. Nonce Glasses tittered nervously; Solitary Guy's eyes looked like they were fixed on an imaginary 18-wheeler driving directly at his head.

'Well, I suppose that's one goal,' deadpanned the psychologist.

'And who the fuck is *this*?' enquired Paul, gesturing vaguely at me.

Suddenly, I could very much see the appeal of hiding behind nonce glasses.

I quickly got the feeling that nobody was more at home in the prison, not the staff, and certainly not me, than Paul was. Meetings in prisons tend to be rather tense, difficult affairs, where the agendas of staff and prisoners come into close conflict, but no matter how tense the meeting Paul just slouched through it, arms folded and a near-constant smirk on his face. Except for those few moments when he sensed he had someone in a compromising

position – then his face would contort with righteous fury, like a televangelist from the Midwest
USA, as he let them know exactly how they now
owed him something and by God was it time for
him to collect.

Outside of prison, Paul had been one of
those individuals who I am probably asked the
most about: a hitman. I am tempted to write
'assassin', but 'assassin' has all sorts of glamorous connotations: what Paul did was not
glamorous in any way. When people owed him
or his bosses money, he would either find them,
tie them up and torture them, or order any of
his spineless yet almost equally brutal under-
lings, driven by a combination of fear and a
desire to become the 'big man' themselves, to
do the same. Paul's reign of terror extended
across several counties in England, aggres-
sively pushing drugs on vulnerable men and
women, backed up by his cronies. Nearly all of
them were also addicted to the crack cocaine
that Paul dealt, giving him nearly absolute
control over their lives.

Finally, things went too far: a rival appeared on the drug scene and started threatening business. Paul gathered several younger accomplices – one of them a boy so young he had to be tried in a youth court – and together they ambushed the other dealer and shot him dead with multiple bullets from a sub-machine gun. At trial, Paul instructed his legal team to blame everything on his young co-defendants, exonerating himself absolutely. After conviction, he used every single appeal attempt allowed to him by the legal system to get this narrative to stick. In a testament to his ongoing power even from inside, the basis of the appeals was that several witnesses to the original trial decided to withdraw their statements or change their stories. Reading through the trial notes, I became deeply impressed with the police who must have moved extremely quickly to secure witness testimony before the apparatus of Paul's klepto-pharmaceutical intimidation machine persuaded them to change their stories. Although it didn't mean a great deal to me at the time, I also saw that Paul had a PCL-R score of 38 out of 40, which meant that he would have been in the most psychopathic 1 per cent of all prisoners.[1]

There are many, many men and women for whom prison is a terrible, terrible place: a place full of restriction, bullying and soul-sapping boredom, where the only constant friends are your own sense of guilt, fear and loneliness. However, for some – and I have never known anyone do this so well as Paul – even the maximum-security jail where we met seemed to be a home away from home.

Paul had been born into a criminal family, inducted by his father at a young age into the 'con code' of never grassing, never showing respect for authority and doing your time without ever cracking. He was also good-looking, with a shock of black hair and great cheekbones, only slightly filled out by the relatively slow, sedate pace of prison life, which meant that people tended to give him more leeway than his terrible criminal past suggested they should. Cons and prison officers of all ranks and levels of the hierarchy almost seem to defer to Paul as though the prison was *his* place, his web into which we had all been pulled by a variety of career choices of varying degrees of questionability.

So, it was into this web that I stepped, fresh out of prison security training, trying to understand what 'power' meant inside institutions and how psychopaths' unique personalities helped or hindered them in such an environment. Paul could not have been nicer to me: he seemed to be in every prisoner meeting I attended for the first week, and also the guitar club where he was a regular attendee well-known for his zealous, if not harmonically faithful, interpretations of Leonard Cohen classics. Sensing I was a bit lost in the new, complicated and highly rigid prison regime, he made several helpful suggestions for sessions I should attend 'if I wanted to know what was really going on in here'. Intrigued, I agreed to attending a number of social and treatment activities around the prison over the next couple of weeks.

Mostly, this was a great success: Paul was always gregarious and keen to integrate me, as well as being popular with the inmates and some – but not all – of the staff. I often wonder what might have happened in the prison were it not for Josie, a five-foot-nothing forensic psychologist who looked like she barely came up to Paul's waist, but absolutely had his number. Whenever she was around, she would take it upon herself to narrate the subtext of Paul's every statement: 'When you say it like that, Paul, it sounds to me a bit like a threat' or 'I don't know why, Paul, but I feel a bit like you're trying to make me look stupid in front of the group. Do you want to explain why that is?' After a while Paul got the message and started being a lot more cautious around Josie.

I came to appreciate the easy-going charm Paul displayed outside of treatment meetings and also his apparent understanding of my naivety and eagerness to understand prison life. Informal groups – cooking classes, playing chess (yes, psychopaths can be great chess players), even just mealtime chats – with Paul present were never dull as there was always some new, interesting dynamic or juicy piece of prison gossip that surprised everyone, sometimes the staff included. One of his favourite topics and sources of mirth was what he called the 'sausage club', an apparently secretive society of sexual transactions that took place between the other prisoners, most of whom self-identified as straight and displayed rampantly homophobic attitudes, but seemed to believe at the same time that sex with other men was better than no sex at all. I say 'apparently' because Paul seemed to know exactly who owed who what sexual favour at any moment, and who was jealous because someone got a blowjob from someone else in the shower on Monday, and so on. He would conclude with a robust disclaimer such as, 'Of course, I don't ever get involved in those prohibited behaviours myself', which I thought was perhaps there to make the staff feel they were doing their jobs a bit, but at the same time I did wonder why someone who gave so little of a shit about anything or what anyone else thought would bother to dissuade them that he was doing anything untoward.

While this was fun to begin with, the more time I spent listening to Paul the more I came to respect the prison staff, perhaps especially Josie, in their handling of this exceptionally difficult group of men. I also began to see that, far from making everyone's difficult life more enjoyable with a 'bit of banter', Paul was effectively spreading poison around the institution: selectively releasing rumour and innuendo to keep the staff on their toes and the prisoners too concerned about their illicit antics being revealed to ever challenge him.

Of course, in time, I became the victim of one of Paul's manufactured dramas.

One of the biggest challenges for me as a non-prison officer within the prison was trying to get access to the things that happened outside the experience of the prison's clinical staff, who were mainly on a nine-to-five shift. Life in the prison for 'civilian' staff was a fairly safe and often mundane experience, much like any other job. However, we regularly came to the morning briefing to hear tales of the horrors that had happened during the evening and night shifts, while we were all safe at home. I had decided that the only way to really understand this was to do an 'A' shift; to spend a full 12-hour shift in the prison, 7am to 7pm, and experience what the officers and prisoners did when we weren't there. This would take some planning on my part: for starters, I was in my mid-twenties and not particularly given to 6am rises. Second, I would need to fill up my day so that I was neither too bored nor too tired to make sense of what was going on. I asked Paul for advice.

'Mate, you need to come along to breakfast and dinner. Everyone's tired and hungry, and that's where the shit really hits the fan.'

For a moment, Paul hesitated, apparently thinking about something. This was uncommon for him.

'You also got to come to the wing business meeting, that's at 2pm: and the men talking group, that's at 4, I'm in that. There's the treatment session that runs every day, too: that's really important for you to come to. Are you writing this down?'

Yes, as it turns out, I was. I was also taking the advice of this apparently sincere, very psychopathic man quite seriously, perhaps too seriously.

My 'A' shift went as well as can be expected: I got up early, came to breakfast and watched semi-serious rows break out over portion sizes. I learned about the 'phantom shitter' who fouled the showers every morning, and I was introduced to another inmate, Patrick, who had a kind of insult diarrhoea, where he couldn't help but produce blood-curdling dismissals of staff and prisoners at the slightest provocation, delivered so loud and fast that the individual words were indistinguishable. 'Fuckyourmotherhopeshe dieso'arsecancer' was a memorable but relatively low-key example. I attended all the security briefings as staff handed over important information about safety between night and morning shifts, then again the next day; and interviewed a couple of prisoners about their particularly upsetting criminal history, one of which involved burning someone to death in a car. It was very hard work, and when I got back to my cold, rented flat at 7.40pm I sat down and fell straight asleep before I'd even managed to type up my notes from the day.

It wasn't until the next day when I attended the treatment orientation group, as usual, with a mix of officers, civilian staff and prisoners, that I had the slightest idea something was not right.

Paul was there and apparently very, very offended about something.

'Fuck were you yesterday?' He was looking directly at me.

'Err, what ... I ...'

'You said you'd come to the men talking group.'

I racked my brains: had I said that?

'I was in the treatment session, I thought that was—'

'Nah ... fuck's sake. You're all the same, you lot. I said I was going to be in the men talking group and you said that you'd come to it.'

I was mortified. By the nature of my research project I was there under sufferance of all the staff and prisoners, and if someone thought I had acted unfairly or unethically then my research was all in jeopardy.

'I'm really sorry,' I began. 'I didn't realise ...'

The most menacing sneer I can recall ever seeing crossed Paul's face.

'You mean you thought you'd take the easy option and hang out with the staff when you're supposed to be understanding what life's like for cons. I thought you were better than that, mate.'

I looked around the group, feeling the depth of my shame. Nobody met my gaze. Paul was shaking his head. Louise, the officer who was running the orientation group, had a rueful look on her face. It seemed that everyone was aware that I couldn't be counted on to follow through on my promises. Who was going to trust me now to tell me important stuff so I could do my job? Fuck.

Later that day I managed to get my head back together and realised that I had been played for a fool with one of the oldest tricks in the book. It was the same trick that Richard Pryor's character falls for in *Moving*: give the punter a mass of banter and irrelevant chat to confuse them and hide among it important pieces of information (like where Paul was actually going to be that day) that you reckon they won't pick out of the mix. Honestly, I was more disappointed with myself than cross with Paul; I had become carried away with the idea of understanding the prisoner experience and forgotten that they were there for a reason. After all, if in a situation where Paul was detained against his will and had virtually no power at all he could still make a fool out of a man with a PhD, imagine what he could do in the community if he was allowed to do and say whatever he wanted.

As if to reinforce the point, the next day I tried to avoid Paul as much as possible, but when I finally saw him at guitar club he didn't seem to have any ill will, or indeed any memory of shaming me out of existence the day before. He was genial and charming as ever. Only Louise, the officer, seemed to be notably less warm towards me. She was quite an upstanding character, very neat and upright, and not someone who gave the impression of tolerating infractions easily, so perhaps my technically not wrong but arguably immoral behaviour had displeased her, as did the slightly immature and over-enthusiastic actions of a large group of younger male officers who were based on the same wing.

Later the next week, Paul and I even had a bit of a rebonding session over a shared love for Radiohead's album *OK Computer*. He asked me if I wouldn't mind printing him off some guitar tablature from the internet, maybe for the song 'Lucky' – which just so happened to be both of our favourite tracks from the album – and 'Karma Police' too. Sensing an opportunity to return to Paul's good graces, and perhaps reconnect with his stream of gossip and insider knowledge, that night I dutifully downloaded, printed out and stapled the guitar tabs together, with a bit more care than I might have done if they were for my use.

However, when I got to the prison car park the next day, something made me hesitate. Suddenly the question of whether or not staples were allowed in the prison seemed extremely important and, in the best tradition of criminal justice work, it seemed a better idea not to take the risk. The guitar tablature remained on the seat of my car and I resolved to bring them in later when I'd taken the staples out. Nice and safe.

Fortunately, as it transpired, things didn't quite work out as planned: in the end I had to leave the prison for a few weeks shortly after this, earlier than planned as I had switched my work contracts over. When I came back, I was no longer a university nerd, but employed by the Prison Service as a Lead Researcher, a *bona fide* member of the (civilian) prison staff. In the melee, I had forgotten all about Paul's tabs and they had become lost in the morass of paperwork all academics hefted about across jobs before cloud storage and digitising.

The first day back in the prison, things seemed a little off. Everyone looked very tense and nobody stopped to congratulate me on my new job or even acknowledge me. Something was clearly up, but the prison was running exactly as normal: prisoner movement at 7.50, morning meeting at 8.30, work in the morning, treatment sessions in the afternoon. When I went onto the wing, there were a few new prisoners, which was to be expected as the prison was supposed to be filling up to justify our additional funding from the DSPD programme – and no sign of Paul. That was odd because he had been on the 'lifer' wing where moving was unlikely because so many of the prisoners were perceived as very high-risk offenders with long tariffs (the time before a life-sentenced prisoner is eligible for parole) and/or high levels of psychopathy, like Paul.

Together, this meant that nobody on the ward was particularly high priority for treatment: they were going nowhere fast. So, where had Paul gone? Guitar club was not until the following week, and I saw on the timetable that the treatment orientation group was not running either, so I couldn't ask any of the cons or staff.

It wasn't until much later that day that I finally managed to find Jackie, who had been my colleague since my first days in the prison. She was probably, to paraphrase Francis Ford Coppola's *Apocalypse Now*, wound a bit tightly for any prison, let alone a maximum-security one full of psychopaths, but she was bright, loyal, knew the prison regulations inside out, and had a good ear for gossip, which made her a great companion.

By this time, I had worked in maximum-security settings across the country for a total of almost two years, so I had seen and heard a lot of crazy stuff: security breaches, deaths in custody, terrible self-harm and shocking violence. Still, my jaw dropped as Jackie told the story.

*

The week before there had been a food fight among the rowdy younger officers on the lifer wing. It had been after the prisoners were locked up, so while probably not appropriate for professionals charged with keeping some of the highest-risk men in the country safely detained, this wasn't anything particularly concerning. However, officer Louise had been passing by at the time, seen the mess generated and rightly called the officers out on it, threatening to report them to the senior officer. Most of the officers had taken this in good humour and stopped, but one, perhaps someone who disliked Louise or being told what to do by women, couldn't help firing back: 'Piss off Lou, we know about you and Paul.'

What had he meant? Perhaps nothing would have come of it had Louise not decided to press the issue, which she did probably because she realised that she could not continue to work in the prison if she could not command the respect of her colleagues. However, what came out of it was devastating. When the young male officer was questioned about his comment by the prison management, he – perhaps out of naivety, perhaps because he wanted to do the right thing – broke the code of silence that exists between staff in any big institution about mistakes their colleagues may have made. Louise, he said, was engaged in a relationship with Paul.

I was astonished as more details emerged, contradicting everything I thought I knew about the prison and Louise. The relationship was sexual and had been going on for about two months. It had started some months before that when Louise had agreed to bring Paul a men's magazine – nothing graphically pornographic, just a 'lad's mag'. The next thing had been a compact disc; I thought of the guitar tabs on my car seat, and my blood ran cold and hot with shame and relief that it wasn't me who'd fallen into this spider's web. Then came the real pornography, then cigarettes (all technically permitted but also potentially powerful things for a prisoner to have for trading), incrementally building up to a tiny bit of cannabis. At the same time, Paul dangled little compliments for Louise to pick up, crumbs from the master's table;

even though he was a prisoner, there was no doubt that the other cons were terrified of him and his word carried weight and influence, even with some of the staff who reckoned that keeping Paul sweet meant a quiet life on the ward.

Paul was a genuine manipulator, a Machiavellian who consciously and deliberately used other people to achieve his personal goals. One of the reasons Hannibal Lecter is such a compelling depiction of a psychopath is his ability to manipulate seemingly every situation to his advantage; to extract his 'quid pro quo' from every conversation or interaction. To do this, however, requires a high degree of both intelligence and life experience, and, from what I've seen, most men and women in the criminal justice system lack either of these to even the level of the average person in the street.

Most psychopaths lie, cheat and manipulate in large because their brains are wired from infancy to reach for these tactics in the way that we would reach for basic manners, compliments or humour to get what we need (or think we need). But many of them also do this simply because they have never been shown another way, and the poverty of learning and socialisation in some psychopaths' lives is truly disheartening. While I was working with Paul, I remember an officer telling a prisoner, 'Stop pressing your cell button, Christ, you're like the boy who cried wolf.' The prisoner became furious: he was a grown man in his thirties, not a boy, and, 'What did wolves have to do with anything?' One of the senior officers calmed the prisoner down and told him the fable of the shepherd boy crying wolf. The prisoner was dumbfounded: nobody had ever taken the time to teach him one of the fundamental moral stories of our society.

Paul shows us, however, that there is a darker shade of manipulation than the one that is done simply as a survival tactic. He may not have been Hannibal Lecter but at the same time it certainly seemed that his every word, every act, every shared piece of gossip, was a gift that could be redeemed later to his advantage: everyone was a means to an end. Unfortunately, that very much included Louise.

Gradually, Louise had found herself spending more time with Paul. I thought of the guitar club and therapy sessions and wondered if these were even her genuine interests. I don't know when Paul first made a pass at her or if he even needed to; often it is not the brilliance of the manipulator that makes the difference between falling for their schemes or not, but rather the fact that most people have vulnerabilities that a good manipulator knows how to exploit. I had been naive and eager to please. Louise was too compassionate, too keen to help, which sounds like a bizarre weakness to have, and at the same time too invested in the role of 'rule enforcer' on the prison. Once Paul had persuaded her to bend the rules even once, he knew she could potentially do anything for him because her mind would find a way of 'undoing' the act of rule-breaking by being tougher with the rules; of rationalising that since *she* was the one doing it, and she was making sure all these other rules were being followed, it must have been alright. Of course, this was also her own undoing: she had tried too hard to enforce the rules with her colleagues and they had called her bluff.

At some point, Paul and Louise's relationship had become intimate, which is no small feat in a prison bristling with security cameras and watchful staff with excellent lines of sight. When Louise had a night shift, they had met regularly in the laundry room after bang-up to have sex and – worse yet – she brought in a steady stream of illicit items that Paul could trade with other prisoners, in absolute contravention of prison regulations and her job as a prison officer. But perhaps the worst part was that the two of them had used their relationship to ensure Paul was unchallenged in his dominance over the other prisoners on the wing. He would threaten them with violent repercussions if they found out about the relationship while simultaneously using the threat of staff sanctions through Louise to ensure he benefitted from any trading of luxuries or contraband. It was a racket, with stark similarities to the one Paul had run before being sent to prison, and one of the most respected and apparently upright officers was right at the heart of it.

The consequences of this were devastating for Louise. She lost her job, of course, and was charged with misconduct in public office, which was in a respect quite lucky: had she been a nurse in a secure hospital rather than a prison she could have been charged with sexual relationship with a vulnerable adult. This would have landed her with a jail term and resulted in her being placed on the sex offenders register; a horrible end to a promising professional career. Paul had been transferred to another prison. The officers who had been involved in the ill-fated food fight had not escaped unscathed either: a couple of them had been found to have concealed information pertinent to security relating to the affair and were suspended from their positions without pay. I think the rest probably knew about it too, but prison management couldn't risk suspending many otherwise competent and respected officers.

The impact on morale within the prison had also been tough: everyone was confused that such a respected and apparently upstanding officer could have fallen prey to a psychopath in such a way. No wonder nobody was particularly pleased to see me that day: they were still trying to process all the loss and betrayal they felt. I wondered if anyone was also feeling what I was feeling. I had come very close to giving in to one of Paul's requests to bring material into a prison that – while maybe not against the strict word of the rules – might well have been the 'gateway' into further or more frequent requests. I had made the first step down the dark path of wanting to make a psychopath like me, even though they had shown themselves quite capable of treating me like someone beneath their contempt, and only luck, or perhaps some kind of primal paranoia, had kept me from falling all the way down the rabbit hole of colluding with a prisoner and losing my job. For an arch-Machiavellian like Paul, it had been far too easy to identify my pressure points; I think that his skill was probably most evident in the way he humiliated me in front of other staff and prisoners before offering me a way to 'redeem myself' in his eyes, to become someone he could confide his desires in again.

*

I wish I could say what happened to Louise was a one-off issue, but during the next three years there were three similar incidents at prisons and hospitals across the UK where nurses or prison officers had started a relationship with men in their care. In every case, the patient or prisoner at the centre of the case was a psychopath, and in every case the staff member was found to be the perpetrator of sexual abuse, not a victim, and lost jobs, careers and livelihoods when they were discovered. These incidents still happen, perhaps less frequently, but there was one case reported by the media from Scotland as recently as 2019[2]. These very unfortunate tales remind us of two things: firstly that while psychopaths can be incredibly charming, underlying that charm is always an unreservedly self-serving agenda; and secondly that anywhere there are psychopaths, someone who becomes isolated from their peers, no matter how respected or experienced that person might be, is at risk of being compromised.

Many years later, my supervisor in a secure hospital, a very respected psychoanalyst, would describe this as 'perversion': the psychopath's ability to set up a 'system within a system' that is in direct contradiction to the standards the original system holds. In the case of the prison, this meant to compromise the 'sealed container' of the institution by bringing in contraband and introducing a black economy running beneath the surface; and to find a way to corrupt every person and every standard. Of course, there is also a second, psychoanalytic meaning to 'perversion', which is to take a sexual satisfaction from socially unacceptable desires and behaviours. In all my experience, nobody has bettered Paul in making perversion a reality.

Chapter Three
Tony, The Conman

I first met Tony on the admissions ward of a secure psychiatric hospital on my first day as an NHS employee, working on a project to understand how modern secure psychiatric wards function. Following two months of inductions and training on everything from spotting every form of marijuana currently in production to incapacitating an attacker without leaving a mark, I was permitted to step onto the ward. For me, as for everyone else starting that day, the one thought repeating endlessly in my mind was 'please, *please* let me not cock up and cause a security breach', because, we were told, that would mean our jobs and our careers would be irrevocably over. Not to mention the fact that a dangerous killer or rapist might then escape to victimise the surrounding area as, we were again told, had happened many times before. The single worst security breach, of course, was to allow yourself to be manipulated by a psychopathic patient and compromise the entire hospital.

The ward was a brand new building, still going through some teething pains: the main window in the living space faced west, meaning that even in spring it became uncomfortably hot on a sunny day, which didn't strike me as a good idea in a space for 15 violent psychopaths. The month before I arrived one of the patients had found a way into the crawlspace above and caused significant amounts of damage to the electrical work and piping, as well as huge embarrassment to the hospital management. He had made his way up there using a piece of wood that had been glued to the top of the doorframe to make it safe as a ligature point: that is, so that nobody could use the doorframe to hang themselves. The NHS Trust had promptly moved the patient to another secure hospital where, we were told, he had done almost exactly the same thing, so he'd probably be on his way back fairly soon.

In the middle of this anxious hothouse, where leisurewear-clad patients flopped listless around the ward, there sat a man in a well-fitted charcoal suit, looking the very picture of calm and reading a newspaper. This would be my first time meeting one, or so I thought, as I had only seen them as talking heads on TV, and heard reverent descriptions by security staff, but I knew this man had to be a consultant psychiatrist. The de facto leaders and lynchpins of any psychiatric inpatient service, psychiatrists make the big decisions about who leaves and who stays, who in their minds is 'cured', and who needs to spend more of a potentially unlimited amount of time detained in the hospital. Consultants – the highest grade of psychiatrist – were paid quite considerable sums in those days and could afford such luxuries as tailored suits, undoubtedly looking down on my sociologist's uniform of cotton-and-corduroy. Feeling ill-prepared and insecure, but mindful of my mission to talk to everyone, I reverently approached this reclining figure and introduced myself.

'Hello,' said the psychiatrist, gracing me with a small smile. 'I'm Tony.' Honoured to be acknowledged by such an authority, it was at that point that I noticed Tony wasn't wearing the regulation-issue NHS Trust ID badge that we had all been told was the hospital equivalent of a liver. He must have been terribly important.

'I expect you know who I am,' continued the psychiatrist, 'everyone else around here does.' My anxious stomach did somersaults: evidently that did not include me, which made me worry that I might have already committed a dreaded cock-up already by not knowing this man's name. What rattled me more, however, was the realisation that Tony was not even wearing his key belt. *No keys!* Did he have a security *escort*? Had he been sent by the Department of Health to perform an unannounced inspection of the hospital? Could I possibly be more ignorant?

A nurse appeared at my shoulder. 'Come on, Tony, you know you're not supposed to be wearing that suit after ward round has finished. Anyway, it's bang-up time now, so off you fuck.' Tony glanced at the nurse momentarily, and I thought I saw the mildest trace of anger flash across his face, but then he wearily complied and – with a dramatic sigh – fucked off as requested in the direction of the patients' rooms.

My overworked brain laboured through this new information before assembling the conclusion that Tony was not, in fact, a psychiatrist. Not only was he not a psychiatrist, he was a patient with an extensive history of conning and manipulating others, who was apparently also very effective at looking just like a psychiatrist. I began to think that even my elevated concerns about cocking up were not even close to high enough.

Tony was a relative exception to most of the psychopaths I've met because his early life didn't, on the face of it, sound destitute or abusive. Unlike Paul, he hadn't been born into the kind of criminal life where violence was a necessary part of growing up; and unlike a depressingly large proportion of the other patients I worked with, he hadn't wanted for food or been physically or sexually abused as a child. Instead, Tony's upbringing featured many far more insidious forms of abuse or perversion that it took me a long time to really understand, and I didn't really get it until I had a chance to talk about him with a senior clinician in another service who happened to have worked with him before. So although Tony could be a pompous ass, so much so that occasionally his care team took a kind of vicarious pleasure in watching him squirm under the predatory gaze of the other criminal psychopaths on the ward, I couldn't help sometimes but feel sorry for him. When I found out more about his family life in the following years, this feeling intensified and I often found myself relieved when he did something utterly shitty to one of the patients or reduced a nurse to tears: it helped to remind me that I was dealing with someone who was capable of absolutely terrible behaviour and the most astonishing sexism.

Just as Paul's father had taught him almost everything he knew about violence, crime and aggression, Tony's dad had been an archetypal conman: a Frank Abagnale from *Catch Me If You*

Can, drinking and philandering his way around the world selling incredible things (the Pyramids! London Bridge!) to credulous people at literally unbelievable prices (yours for only £100,000!). His relationship with Tony's mother had been tense and quite insubstantial – after all, what use are a wife and child when you are a metropolitan sales-man and playboy – and after a few years, when Tony was eight, he had simply disappeared. There was some suggestion that Tony's mother did not even know her sometime husband's real name, so talented was he at passing himself off as someone else. Time and Tony's inconsistent recall make it hard to be certain but nevertheless: glibness and superficial charm, multiple 'marital-type' rela-tionships and a propensity for conning others are classic hallmarks of a primary psychopath, the most genetically heritable variant. In other words, Tony's genes certainly had form.

After her husband's disappearance, Tony's bereft and lonely mother invested all her hopes and love into her son, making him in many respects a substitute for her lost husband. In what psychoanalysts would consider a classic case of narcissistic enmeshment,[1] Tony's mother became besotted with him and refused to give him punishment or sanctions, however obnoxious or extreme his behaviour. I always wince inwardly when I read the *Viz* cartoon 'Spoilt Bastard', as the titular character's mother endlessly permits all kinds of awful, self-centred behaviour by her offspring on the basis that as a single mother this is what she has to do to show her love. But this is what Tony experienced, and the result was that he was completely unable to emotionally separate himself from his mother, both in terms of his love for her – I think that is what it was, although often this was indistinguishable from a kind of infinitely jealous indulgence – and in terms of his tendency to simply disregard any kind of boundary any other woman ever asserted for him. This made for a special kind of tension whenever he was allocated a female primary nurse, which was often given that over 80 per cent of nurses are women.

In hospital, Tony's behaviour was a kind of extreme parody of a narcissistic and histrionic personality: both infuriating and yet oddly genial with a great talent for looking crestfallen, which is a lost art these days. Superficially, he was always charming and engaging; wishing everyone a good day, even – particularly – when we obviously weren't having one, and signing up for every optional activity that didn't involve physical exercise. Even when not hamming up the psychiatrist look, Tony was, relatively speaking, very well dressed, eschewing the lazy sportswear sported by the rest of the patient group in favour of a range of patterned shirts and corduroy trousers; he persisted in dressing in this fashion despite the objections of some staff and the ridicule of other patients, which took some gall when your peers included multiple murderers, drug kingpins and serial killers.

When people took the mickey about his posh clothes, Tony tended to respond with almost total indifference, when he even appeared to listen at all. With a deep sigh, he would respond, 'Sticks and stones ...' or some other glib brush-off that was oddly effective at sending a clear message to the other patients: 'I'm sure you think that's very funny, but

I simply don't care what you think.' Tony also had withering put-downs for staff members. One of his favourites being the evergreen, 'I'll take that on board', which, at least the first time you heard it, communicated the chance he might actually be listening to what you were saying, and a superficial openness to change. The problem was, for anyone living or working with Tony, that the charm rapidly wore off at the second and third times you heard one of his glib responses or hollow compliments. 'You're the only person here who ever listens to me,' he once told me, 'I feel I can be honest with you, but I just can't trust the other staff.' Powerful stuff, perhaps, until I learned he had said the exact same thing to at least three other staff in the hospital.

Tony also stood out because he had a wide vocabulary and could give a good impression of listening, but you quickly noticed that this 'listening' was actually the ability to wait patiently for you to stop speaking so that he could speak more, apparently not having paid the slightest bit of attention to what you had said. Rather, he would pick up

some key words from the conversation and dan-
gle these in front of you to give the impression of
being deeply interested, while actually serving his
own agenda. I remember a conversation that went
something like this:

'Good morning Tony.'

'Good morning to you, Mark. You know I was
thinking about something you said yesterday
about social anthropology?'

'Oh, really? I—'

'Yes, I was thinking about how superior that
way of thinking is to the way the psychologists
think around here. You know, we really are products of our social environments, aren't we?'

In this exchange, Tony was using something
I had mentioned to him about culturally context-
ual ways of understanding mental illness and
used it to leverage his long-standing beef about
the way he had been, in his view, misunderstood
and mistreated by psychologists and psychiatrists.
Anything I said was only of interest to him in
so far as it directly served his own interests and
worldview. Now you might be thinking, 'Oh well,

that reminds me of my friend/father/uncle/myself",
and I know that all of us tend to select information
that supports our worldview. Imagine, though, if
you did this without ever spending a moment to
listen to someone else's opinions just out of courtesy. Imagine if you didn't even feel the need to
acknowledge that they might be more interesting
than you. This is the blessing and the curse of the
psychopath: other people and their opinions aren't
even worth investing courtesy into.

Another bizarre habit Tony had was describing
situations of a wildly implausible nature and making continual reference to his family's considerable
wealth and to his scholarship in the areas of genetics and ancestry, specifically of British monarchs.
In one exchange that really did my head in, Tony
once told me, quite soon after we met, that he had
written a 13-volume set of biographies of kings of
England from William the Conqueror to Richard II.
I asked him if it had been published and he said
that the manuscript was 'with his publisher' and
they were 'waiting for the right time to release it'.

What made this exchange so bizarre was that Tony was clearly lying. I knew he was lying, he presumably knew that I knew that he was lying, but I couldn't bring myself to challenge the lie. This was not because I was worried about Tony's response – I've found that primary psychopaths are remarkably hard to anger – but because there wasn't any point. If I'd challenged him on it, Tony would simply have amended his lie to keep up with my questioning. The conversation played out in my head:

'Can I read it?'

'No, as I've told you, unfortunately the manuscript is with the publisher, and they won't let me have a computer in here.'

'Umm ... but, how did you write an 800,000-word book if you didn't have a computer?'

'Well, I was allowed one in prison.' (Unlikely but impossible for me to check.)

'How did you deal with the controversy about the accession of Queen Matilda in 1141?'

'Oh, such a minor character – I simply elected to write her out of existence.'

Lies explained by technicalities of regulations and simple bad scholarship make for a tiresome and unsatisfying conversation that I just didn't want to have. So I never did get to the bottom of the history of British kings ... but then I still haven't seen it available for sale in any bookshop. At the time, it was like we both accepted the lie of the book for the fiction it was but pretended that it was true just because, for me, challenging it was too much hard work. Again, there's something quite perverse about this and it reminds me in hindsight of the way that a well known business in the USA refused to pay small invoices to suppliers by simply pretending that they aren't there: daring the supplier to launch a lawsuit, knowing that the cost of such an action would likely exceed the reward.

Hopefully you have got the impression of Tony as someone who was very frustrating to work with, but also that interactions with him could be thought-provoking and that it was very possible to learn something about yourself. Whether this was the limits of your patience with fellow humans, your energy to either challenge or live with obvious lies, or your ability to feel sympathy when the person you are speaking with is so terribly unsympathetic. However, a lot of these feelings changed when I learned how and why Tony had come into the criminal justice system in the first place.

It seemed that Tony had made it his objective in life to become a more effective version of his father, the international playboy conman. Fuelled by emotional and financial support from his mother, Tony stylised himself just as his father had, establishing a network of companies selling fraudulent products and Ponzi schemes, and even established his own credit union for moving money around. It was difficult to establish from Tony exactly how successful these schemes were, but certainly by the time he was first imprisoned he had staff on his payroll and enough cash to finance a lavish lifestyle. Often, while at large in the community he would introduce himself as a South African businessman, the son of a diamond mining family, and given his curiously unplaceable accent and expensive clothing this would have seemed plausible.

However, in one part of his lifestyle Tony differed considerably from most psychopaths. Psychopathic men tend to inveigle themselves into highly unequal, 'marital-type' relationships, usually taken to mean relationships lasting six months or more, where they are parasitic upon their would-be spouse for money and emotional support. Of course, most of these men are also serially unfaithful, but they will generally stick around as long as they can under the pretence of commitment. But Tony was different: perhaps because of his absolute commitment to his mother, he never spoke about ever having had a 'real' relationship: instead, he had preferred casual sex with male sex workers. With his conspicuous apparent wealth, he would cruise the bars and gay red light districts of UK cities and approach male sex workers he'd taken a liking to and offer them extra money for an overnight stay. Knowing the power imbalances present in any sex worker encounter, this must have been a difficult offer to resist: I almost think of Jack the Ripper offering grapes – almost an unimaginable luxury to eighteenth-century sex workers – to his victims to entice them in.

On the day of his index offence (that is, the crime for which he would go to prison), Tony picked up a young, male sex worker and brought him back to a hotel room. He offered him additional money for what he presented as 'light BDSM', to which he agreed: but what Tony had in mind was a series of brutal, sadistic punishments not mentioned in the agreement, ranging from whipping to brutal sexual abuse. When the ordeal was finished, his victim bleeding, bruised and unconscious, Tony left, dropping a cheque for the agreed amount – using his own credit union's chequebook – on the ground in the hotel room.

What happened next is the subject of some dispute but the version I heard from Tony's social worker is that the sex worker, after being released from hospital the next day, went to pay in the cheque only to find that it then bounced. Not, it turns out, because it was fraudulent – although that would not have surprised anyone involved – but rather because Tony had simply forgotten to pay money into the relevant account. Complacency, apathy, callousness, disinterest or just a mistake: all possible interpretations and ones that Tony was never willing to shed any light on. The victim went to the police and was able to give a very detailed description of Tony and his clothes, which were highly visible in the small Midlands town where Tony had chosen to commit his crime: he was arrested and charged within two weeks. The whole offence was so blatant, so flagrant in its abuse of the law and absolute contempt for sex workers, the police and a society that would accept his crooked cheques, that it often crossed my mind that maybe some part of Tony's unconscious wanted him to be caught. But perhaps his narcissistic fantasy had overtaken him to the point where he genuinely thought he was untouchable.

Tony was a one-off even among psychopaths. He had no history of violent convictions before his index offence, although of course the possibility remains open that he had many other victims who never went to the police or who simply fell into the

95 per cent of sexual assault cases (or in 2018, 98 per cent[2]) that never make it to prosecution. One of the other men in the hospital once referred to him as a 'cellophane psychopath', a phrase that I have pondered for a long time since, but have taken to mean that Tony was all 'primary' psychopath: he wasn't really antisocial and he had no 'street cred' or aggression to him. Rather, Tony's personality was like cellophane: a tissue thin, reflective mask that he could rip, change or just dispose of depending on the situation. Getting to know 'the true Tony' often felt impossible, as though a cellophane wrapping insulated him, making him slippery to the touch, and I think the other patients understood this.

Sometimes I wondered if Tony was even a psychopath at all, or just a very extreme version of a narcissist, someone with narcissistic personality disorder like Brian Blackwell. Blackwell was convicted in 2005 of murdering his parents after they discovered he was using their identities to build up tens of thousands of credit card debt in order to pass himself off as an international playboy. However, Blackwell's crime was far more simplistic in many ways: he was narcissistically wounded by his parents' uncovering of his fraud and destroyed them to remove the source of the wound. Something about Tony's offending felt more sadistic; as if it was reliving a much deeper, more perverse sense of injustice that was somehow recreating his relationship with his parents: a mother who was submissive just as a sex worker could be paid to be, and a father who represented the endless wealth and potency Tony pretended to have. So when the cellophane was ripped, what truly lay underneath was not the suave cosmopolitan he presented, but something far darker; something that I don't think any of us except his victims was ever allowed to see.

Chapter Four
Jason, The Liar

My wife likes to keep Radio 6 Music on in the kitchen: it keeps us company in the morning when the kids wake us up before 7am and when we're cooking dinner later in the day, the playlist is sometimes even acceptable. It was a Sunday afternoon in 2014 and I was cleaning up after lunch. Some insipid indie track had wound to its conclusion and the BBC newscaster's reassuringly stentorian tones came on with the day's stories.

'A British man has been found guilty in Italy of murder and attempted murder following a three-week crime spree in early 2013.'

For some reason this tragic but not exceptional piece of news piqued my interest. 'Jason Marshall,' intoned the newsreader, 'was sentenced to 14 years by an Italian court for the murder of a 67-year-old Italian man …'

Wait a moment, I thought: Jason Marshall? I know that name ... yes, he was the guy that absconded from the hospital I worked in a few years back. Wasn't he supposed to be low risk? How could this have happened?

I am going to take a different approach in this chapter and talk about Jason Marshall's case from outside my own experience; one where the information is freely available in the public domain for anyone to review. In this respect, this puts me in the reader's shoes in following the trail of evidence to think about whether a story widely reported in the media might represent a case of psychopathic disorder. As you will see, often there are contradictory details and pieces of information that suggest different possible explanations for someone's behaviour, and some pieces of information don't seem to make sense in any context. This is entirely normal, even – or perhaps especially – for a forensic psychiatrist or psychologist. Very often these professionals draw conclusions on a 'balance of probabilities' rather than outright certainties.

I want to describe this case specifically because it makes an interesting counterpoint to Paul and Tony's stories. These were two men who personified key aspects of the criminal psychopath: a violent, manipulative bully who used the threat of violence to intimidate and control others, and a superficially charming and well-presented yet deeply sadistic fraudster who believed everyone was a plaything for the realisation of his infantile fantasies. This chapter brings to light an aspect of psychopathy that is key but has so far been discussed only tangentially: pathological lying. The case of Jason Marshall demonstrates how this trait makes psychopaths so difficult to work with and estimating their dangerousness such a challenge. Sometimes they appear to wear so many masks – so many identities, so many lies, so many primitive desires. Marshall used lies to construct an identity that justified and excused his behaviour; rejecting and revising them when convenient to the point where the reality was impossible to discern.

Jason Marshall was born in 1989 in East Ham, an area of east London that at the time was one of the most deprived areas in all of Europe. His story sounds depressingly familiar to me, having met a lot of men in prisons and secure hospitals: his parents were heroin addicts and when Marshall was aged ten they were convicted of drug-related crimes and sent to prison. There is not a lot of reliable information about his next few years, although Marshall has given accounts that suggest he moved to Southend, the coastal Essex town, and as a teenager worked as a male escort, usually for older men. Around this time, bereft of clear role models and in and out of contact with the care system, he has also said he started to use fancy dress costumes to pose as people in positions of authority: police officers, air cadets, park attendants and, perhaps most worryingly, a nurse.

Impersonation and fraud, such as we saw Tony engage in during the previous chapter, are aspects of 'primary' psychopathy. Usually this impersonation serves a clear material purpose for the psychopath, whether that is to obtain money or favours. In Marshall's case it is not immediately clear why he assumed these multiple identities.

Sometimes he would board trains posing as a member of the British Transport Police and issue bogus fines to people without tickets, and once he stole police radios from a station when in costume, but there is no indication that he ever collected the fake fines or obtained any material benefit from his actions. Perhaps he simply liked the sense of control that came from playing these socially powerful roles; liked to intimidate other people from a position of strength.

In 2006, Jason's behaviour became known to the police. He had brought a 'sniffer dog' with him while checking fines on the Tube, and London Underground officials had become suspicious because the dog was a Yorkshire terrier – a small and somewhat delicate breed never used in professional work. Marshall was arrested and convicted of robbery, impersonating a police officer and possession of an air rifle in a public place. He did not do well in prison, deliberately harming himself, and in 2008 he was transferred to a medium-security hospital – that is, a psychiatric hospital with only one gate from which unauthorised entry or departure is nearly impossible – for treatment for personality disorder. After two years he was given unescorted leave, which is usually a positive sign that treatment is progressing. However, a few weeks into the privilege he failed to return from an unescorted trip. Medium-security regulations meant that the police had to be informed, and Marshall was returned to prison within a few weeks to serve out the remainder of his sentence.

The *Hackney Gazette*, the secure unit's local paper, had something of a '20/20 hindsight epiphany' after one of his subsequent, serious convictions, in 2017. They alleged failings in management, claiming that the service treating him had been ineffective. Why, they said, wasn't this case of a convicted man absconding from a secure hospital service for psychopaths taken more seriously? Or, more directly: why did nobody see what was coming after this?

The answer to this is a complicated one and it goes beyond the issue of psychopathy into how we understand the 'risk' of reoffending in criminology and forensic psychology. Essentially, reoffending risk is all about rehabilitation: about seeing how effectively someone's past crimes can be rehabilitated to prevent future crimes. At high levels of risk, where crimes are more serious or rehabilitation has failed previously, more precaution is taken because the stakes are higher: but at low levels of risk, especially where a convict has a short offending history, all the models and algorithms suggest the likelihood of reconviction is low. Since around 24 per cent of mental health service users have a criminal record,[1] and nearly a sixth of people in the UK have a mental disorder, the implications of trying to simply treat everyone with a conviction as high risk are massive: over 2.5 million beds would be needed. This means that distinctions need to be made, and in Marshall's case, the judgement of the Ministry of Justice was that the number and severity of his offences would class him as low risk by just about any standard, meaning he could serve out his sentence in prison and there would be no justification for a further expensive intervention such as hospital.

The problem was that – as one former nurse working for the service speaking to the *Gazette* put it, again with the glorious clarity of hindsight – '[i]t was the return to prison that caused [Marshall] to disappear into the system, and his risk to the public to be lost.' Marshall was picked up by the police and was back in prison within three weeks, where he finished his sentence and was released to the community. Of course, what nobody up to this point had realised was how deep and dark his fantasy life truly was, and how the impersonations and elaborate costumes were just that: a dress rehearsal for what was to come.

After his release from prison in 2010, Marshall did not cope well with life in the community. He started drinking and using drugs heavily: a risky combination especially mixed with the psychiatric medication he was already taking. There was a brief period of stability around the London Olympics of 2012, where he was given a regular job as a street cleaner by Newham Council; but after the Olympic hubbub subsided and the clean-up was done, Marshall was made redundant and apparently began to abuse substances even more heavily than before. However, there were no more convictions so nobody – police, professionals or the press – had any inkling of what was about to happen.

It was in early February 2013 when the neighbours of Umberto Gismondi heard loud thumps and screams coming from his flat in Rome. They rushed over to find the 55-year-old man severely bruised and covered in blood, only repeating the name 'Jason Marshall' over and over. When the ambulance arrived, the medics found he had been tied up, gagged, beaten, sprayed with pepper spray and partially suffocated with a pillow. It was possibly a robbery or could have been – since the attacker had been interrupted – something more insidious. The police attending the scene were confused: why would an Italian victim be giving a British-sounding name? And if indeed the attacker was British, how could someone capable of such a serious assault not have been identified by the British police and highlighted as a risk when he came into Italy?

Italian police checking Sr Gismondi's phone found that he had been exchanging messages with someone named 'Gabriel' over the Badoo social networking app, which was a popular dating site, particularly for gay men, before Grindr and Tinder colonised the market. The police reasoned that 'Gabriel' and 'Jason Marshall' must be related, so used the signal from 'Gabriel's' mobile phone through the Badoo app to track him to a bus in central Rome.

Once Marshall was in custody, police realised that an unsolved murder case from 26 January, just four weeks prior to his arrest, had some remarkable similarities to the attack on Sr Gismondi.

Vincenzo Iale, a 67-year-old Italian man living in Torvaianica, just south of Rome, had been found dead in his apartment having been strangled with electrical cord, stabbed dozens of times then left to die, naked, in his own blood. The attacker had then taken Sr Iale's cash card and used it to withdraw €2,000 from a cash machine; the police believed he had been tortured to divulge the PIN number. When police checked Sr Iale's phone, they found details of an arranged meeting with 'Gabriel' over the Badoo dating app. The police thought they might have found the hallmarks of a modus operandi (MO), that is a 'signature' method of committing crime, associated with a would-be serial killer. Marshall was charged with murder and attempted murder.

Details of the trial available in English are quite scant, but they sound chaotic. Marshall complained that the process was taking too long, breaching his human rights, and repeatedly interrupted proceedings to claim he was 'the Archangel Gabriel, messenger of God' and 'here to deliver a prophecy'. He claimed a third party, a male prostitute called 'Michael' – a congruently biblical choice of scapegoat – had murdered Sr Iale in front of him. No evidence of this was offered to the court, however.

Marshall probably knew that delusional thinking about biblical characters can be characteristic of people with a psychotic illness, rather than psychopathy, and may also have known that Italian law states that people with a mental illness are eligible for shorter sentences than those without. In the case of murder, a life sentence can be imposed without eligibility for parole for 26 years. A psychiatrist appointed by the court suggested a long list of diagnoses for Marshall: psychotic disorder, delusions, Asperger's syndrome and borderline personality disorder. In the end the judge partly upheld the mental illness narrative and sentenced Marshall to 16 years in an Italian prison – considerably below the maximum he could have imposed.

All of this is certainly strange and disturbing enough. However, it wasn't until a year after Marshall's conviction for murder in Italy that the story became darker yet. Peter Fasoli, a computer repairman living in Northolt, north-west London, had been found dead by British police in his burned-out apartment in January 2013. The fire brigade had investigated at the time and concluded that the fire had started on the bed, which was made of highly flammable material. Likely it was started due to a faulty light and was nothing beyond a tragic accident. As part of procedure, they referred the case to the Crown Prosecution

Service, who also ruled the death as not suspicious and took no further action. It wasn't until after the conclusion of the inquiry, when his remaining possessions including his burned but functional laptop had been returned to his family, that his nephew, Christopher, discovered footage of a number of sexual encounters that Mr Fasoli had recorded. Most of them were innocuous if somewhat surprising to his family, who had described him as a loner, but the final video, recorded on the night of the fire, must have been at once horrific and devastating to watch.

In the eight-hour video, images of which are now well-distributed on the internet, Jason Marshall is seen entering Mr Fasoli's flat posing as an "undercover policeman", but actually wearing a t-shirt and a fake US police badge and gun holster, and again calling himself Gabriel. The two chat for a while, with Marshall demanding cake, coffee and classical music and describing his 'dirty work' for MI5. The two play this out as if it were a sexual fantasy, and it does seem to be that, until Marshall asks Mr Fasoli to undress for his massage, at which point, perhaps mercifully, the laptop camera is deactivated. The audio continued to record. Marshall then then mock 'arrests' Mr Fasoli, tying him up by the hands and feet and – with what now seems like terrible inevitability – gagging him. The recording suggests that this starts out as part of the game but rapidly turns dark, with Mr Fasoli asking how he would know for sure whether this was 'for real'; after that there are sounds of him choking, then of someone searching the apartment, spreading around what sounds like a liquid and finally the horrifying 'click' of a lighter. Marshall had apparently murdered Mr Fasoli in cold blood under the pretence of sex, then robbed him and set fire to the apartment to destroy the evidence; and he had got away with it for nearly two years, partly by fleeing to Italy using his victim's stolen money.

Presented with this new evidence the CPS re-opened the enquiry, but because Marshall had no further UK record it wasn't until January 2017 that the link with the Iale and Gismondi attacks was made and a European arrest warrant was issued for Marshall's return to the UK to be tried for Peter Fasoli's murder. Again, when this case came to trial in July 2017, there was little to help us understand Marshall's motives. Contradicting evidence given in Rome, Marshall said that he had been so far under the influence of drink and drugs that he did not remember any of the attack. When the prosecutor asked why him why he could remember the Iale murder, he responded that his Italian lawyer had told him not to use this defence as it was a poor one and he should come up with something better. Eventually in Italy he had chosen to rely on 'as if' dream diaries from his court-ordered psychiatry sessions, where he had told a court psychiatrist, in an OJ Simpson-like way, how he would have committed a murder. Under oath in the British court, Marshall claimed that 'I wasn't under oath in the Italian court, and when I swear an oath to God I will never lie, I would rather die', which to me achieves the remarkable feat of mocking both the British and Italian legal systems at the same time.

At sentencing, the judge was predictably ex-coriating of the police and CPS decision not to thoroughly investigate the fire in Mr Fasoli's flat and also to follow due diligence in checking the dead person's social media accounts, which would of course have revealed his planned visitor that evening. Recognising that he was dealing with a serial killer, he imposed upon Marshall a sentence of 39 years to be served in a UK prison. As a British citizen, his time would be served consecutively with his Italian sentence, but would last much, much longer.

I have read a lot of disturbing accounts of assaults, stabbings, murders and rapes in the course of my work, but there is something uniquely distasteful about Marshall's offending against vulnerable older men. Part of this, I think, is that he was so callous about his responsibility: he claimed to have forgotten the crimes under the influence of drugs. This can happen when people commit crimes so terrible that they have 'traumatised' themselves into amnesia, but Marshall's were not random acts of rage: they were carefully planned and effectively executed murders and attempted murders.

The final attack ended only when Marshall apparently selected a victim who was too powerful for him to overcome. People who are truly psychotic, those suffering from paranoid schizophrenia for example, are seldom so instrumental in their attacks and certainly not capable of the level of planning and theatre (costumes, fake identities, sex games) inherent in Marshall's crimes. Since we are dealing with someone for whom fantasy and reality are unusually connected realms, and for whom telling the truth is not something necessary or even helpful, he probably views the rest of us as unworthy or unable of judging him, meaning any explanation he gives us will have to suffice. 'I'll tell them what they deserve to hear.'

Because we don't have access to Marshall's psychiatric files or a copy of his sentencing records, we should be cautious in describing him as a psychopath. Court reports described him as having a 'psychopathic disorder' but this is sometimes used as an old British legal technical term for any disorder involving 'abnormally aggressive or seriously irresponsible conduct',[2] and we don't have a PCL-R

or any other piece of firm evidence to substanti-
ate him being a psychopath. Several psychiatric
reports commissioned by the court at his UK trial
have suggested he may have had a diagnosis of
Asperger's syndrome: a term, no longer used, for
a high-functioning form of autistic spectrum disorder, which has no links to criminal behaviour.
However, since Marshall was detained in a 'severe
personality disorder' unit rather than a specialist
hospital for offenders with autism, it is likely that
psychiatrists believed that a personality disorder, such as psychopathy or antisocial personality
disorder, was the most plausible explanation for
his offending behaviour. The nature of Marshall's
lying – consistent and apparently without shame,
perspective or remorse – has been shown to be
incompatible with a diagnosis of autism. Children with autism show a high degree of what is
called 'semantic leakage' – that is to say, they
may be able to tell a simple lie initially, but their
subsequent defence of the lie will show obvious
inconsistencies.[3] Pathological lying, on the other
hand, of the type present in psychopaths, is very

much about the ability to blend lies seamlessly into one another.

Just as Marshall was able to move from identity to identity, whether as a powerful MI5 operative, then a sex worker, then serial killer, then someone who lost his memory, pathological lying conveys that the psychopath is simply unable to tell the truth for lying, to the point where the liar forgets what the actual truth is. Why might this be? The research evidence is still fairly threadbare, but neuroscientists think that lying is essentially a skill; one that you need to practise to become good at. Psychopaths find it easier to lie generally and 'learn' how to lie more quickly;[4] we think this is because of the differences to the amygdala region of their brain, which is strongly related to 'lying skill'. An active amygdala in a non-psychopath goes into overdrive, sending out a lot of emotion-related signals, possibly shame. In a psychopath, however, the amygdala is underactive from the start and more quickly 'learns' to give a more muted response to lying over time.[5] So, in Marshall's case, his early deception in presenting himself as someone he was

not – a ticket inspector, policeman or park attend-
ant – eventually meant that he was able to assert
any identity he wished with confidence, including
spies and biblical figures.

For me, what sticks out about Jason Marshall's
case is not his diagnosis, or his possible psychopathy, but rather what he did: that he used people's
reliance on truth and honesty – something that,
I hope, is still our default expectation of people
– against them in such a ruthless way. For our soci-
eties to function, we must trust people in uniform
to use their power fairly, we must trust medics to
be appropriately qualified, and when we allow
people to become intimate with us, we trust them
not to abuse that intimacy or our vulnerability
that comes with it. In the same way, any psychiatrist treating a patient will sooner or later have to
trust them to make good decisions for themselves;
and any court expects the accused – under oath or
not – to tell their truth.

Whatever his motives, Jason Marshall exploited all this trust, whether his victims (and not just
the men he killed), his psychiatrists, the police or

the courts, in a way that displayed nothing but absolute contempt for their gullibility. It is chilling to think about how any person could be so absolutely alienated from this fundamental social understanding; for me, it shows how people's absolute refusal to be accountable for their actions beckons the end of our civilisation.

Chapter Five
Arthur, The Parasite

When I was a young boy, my dad, up to that point an academic with a respectable but not exceptional role at a red-brick university, was offered a position in the West Indies through the Commonwealth Secretariat, a government body that supports former British colonies with, among other things, expert policy input. My father thought this was the chance of a lifetime for his family as well as his career, so we all upped sticks and moved to the West Indies. If this sounds to you like an idyllic childhood full of sun, sea and sand then you'd be right: it was paradise. Except for one thing: the place was full of bugs and spiders, a fair proportion of which have no problem biting humans. And I *hated* bugs and spiders even before we moved out there, a situation that the foot-long poisonous centipede trapped, still wriggling, in our kitchen window on the day we arrived did not much ameliorate. Still, I survived all of these hardships and after moving back to the UK, do still pluck up the courage to visit my parents out there occasionally.

Now I'm sure that my dislike of bugs is irrational, but every time I think I'm over it the Universe gives me just enough of a reminder not to give up on the bug-hate just yet. Case in point being just last year, when a family friend in the West Indies was cleaning his house and was bitten on the face by a brown recluse spider. This is a rare occurrence: recluse spiders are not indigenous to the Caribbean and are – as per the name – very reclusive by nature, but the wound had made him terribly sick and left a very nasty (if glamorous) scar on his face. I had never heard of anything like this happening before, so as a serious and committed arachnophobe immediately went about researching recluse bites on the internet. Of course, I was trying to ensure nothing like that could ever happen to me, right?

What I found out really surprised me as it went against some of my worst fears and preconceptions about spiders: recluses, like most spiders, are not capable of simply walking up and biting you, as their fangs can't break human skin. Rather, you must somehow apply counter-pressure to them that forces their fangs into your skin, say by stepping on them, or, in our friend's case, by slapping them as they are crawling away across your face, probably as fast as possible in order to get away from you. It occurred to me that, for every offender I have worked with like Paul (in chapter two), who seek out trouble and seem to relish it, there is another one for whom the offence seems to be a sort of 'perfect storm' of difficult circumstances combined with very, very bad luck: like a kind of social counter-pressure.

My memory has no better illustration of this than Arthur. In many respects I believe that Arthur sought to avoid trouble wherever he could. In fact, I think that perennially avoiding everything – responsibility, accountability, maturity – that would normally be expected to keep him out of trouble seemed to have the opposite effect in his case. Nature abhors a vacuum, perhaps.

I first met Arthur in prison very shortly after starting my first job there, while I was still wondering if Paul was out to help me or destroy me. Unlike with Paul, however, I can scarcely recall my early interactions with Arthur; I just know I must have met him because I have the notes from a case meeting where both our names are clearly listed. Although I can remember the meeting and the attending staff, I don't remember Arthur being there at all. I don't think he can have said much, if anything. If he did, I can't remember his voice, whether it was high or low, fast or slow, baritone or alto. He was the essence of non-remarkability.

Perhaps because of that, the prospect of writing about Arthur did not initially fill me with much enthusiasm. When I decided that I wanted to write this chapter, I realised I had completely forgotten his real name and had to search through my notes to find it. In some respects, that should make writing about him straightforward: after all, Arthur is not someone whose (real) name or the details of his crime received much attention in the press. In fact, it's unlikely that anyone outside Arthur's family and the police and prison officers who dealt with his case has any idea who he is. Even in person, he is almost like a shadow personified: short, stick-thin and a shade of crepuscular grey that it doesn't quite look possible for a human being to be. If I saw him again today on the street, I don't think there is any chance I would recognise him, whereas I could pick out Paul or Tony in an instant. In other words, Arthur is barely there; and perhaps that is a very important thing to know in order to understand why he was so dangerous.

The Psychopathy Checklist contains a number of odd items, but at least one seems to feature a strong value judgement: 'Parasitic Lifestyle', which is defined as: 'An intentional, manipulative, selfish, and exploitative financial dependence on others as reflected in a lack of motivation, low self-discipline, and inability to begin or complete responsibilities.' People who meet the criteria for this trait tend to be in relationships where they have carefully cho-sen friends or partners who can either be charmed or bullied into supporting all the patient's material needs, whether for money, food, drugs, booze or even (in one case) designer clothes. The parasitic psychopath never feels any shame or remorse for this dependency, although they might fake it and promise to change just to keep the status quo, so it will continue indefinitely until they become bored, find a better mark for their parasitism or get themselves arrested.

Arthur was one of three children, having an older brother and sister. His parents had a troubled relationship and were heavy drug users, and although perhaps nothing in Arthur's history stated that he was abused, there is a suggestion that his siblings had a much worse time of it. Either way, when Arthur was ten his father left, permanently, and his brother and sister followed his cue, moving out of the family home and creating their own families and lives. This left Arthur alone with his mother, an arrangement that he found quite cosy; in fact a little too cosy, because after leaving school at 16 Arthur showed no real interest in anything besides sitting around watching TV and prevailing on his mother to cook and clean for him. He wasn't a troublesome youth: he never got into any scrapes as far as I was aware, but neither did he really accomplish much in the way of life. He told me he had some friends that he would hang out with at the park, smoking cigarettes and occasionally playing football. But surely the point of friends is that we speak fondly of them? Arthur never even offered me a single name or adjective about any one of his friends.

Then, when Arthur was just 17, the unthinkable happened: his mother died very unexpectedly of a brain aneurysm. He had been completely dependent on her and was suddenly, completely, on his own. He had no job, few qualifications and very little interest in anything. His brother offered to take him in on a short-term basis, so Arthur moved into a spare room in the house he shared with his girlfriend and tried to get a job so that he could contribute to the rent. For a while, this was successful: he got a job in a kitchen as a potwash and started paying some rent and occasionally buying some groceries. When I spoke to Arthur about this, he said that he had lost the job after three months for showing up late to work too often, but he couldn't understand why this frustrated his brother so much. After all, he'd contributed to the rent already, hadn't he? The idea that rent is a constant expense didn't seem to occur to him, and neither did he seem much to care about the cost of shopping and cooking.

Signed on to unemployment benefit and sitting around the flat all day watching TV and drinking beer, it is not surprising that tensions between Arthur, his brother and – in particular – his brother's girlfriend started to escalate. Matters were made worse by the fact that the girlfriend had now become a fiancée, and they understandably wanted some space of their own. Again, Arthur was completely perplexed by this when I spoke to him about it. 'I didn't cause no trouble around the place,' he asserted, 'just minded my own business.' I don't know many couples in a position to be married who appreciate a family member colonising their living space at all, let alone one who does not cook, go out, pay rent or even shop with any regularity.

Eventually tensions boiled over and Arthur was given his marching orders: aged 18, he had to move out of his brother's house and find somewhere to live on his own. So, he packed a bag and left, but lacking any 'real world' skills he wasn't able to navigate the process of getting a home from the council, and he had no friends he knew well enough to put him up. Almost by default, Arthur became street homeless and started using drugs and drinking heavily. He also began to get in trouble with the police, racking up charges for petty crimes: drunk and disorderly, possession of drugs and burglary. Eventually he got into a fight with someone over a drug debt and the police charged him with a more serious offence of actual bodily harm (ABH) and contacted his brother to bail him out. He reluctantly complied, but was upset by the ragged, shambling mess Arthur had become after six months on the street and brought him back into his flat to live with him and his now-wife.

However, none of the difficulties present in Arthur's previous stay had gone away, and now he was drinking much more heavily and using cannabis and heroin whenever he could get them. This made him unpredictable and quick to anger. Later, working with Arthur in prison, I never quite knew what was going to make him agitated and hostile, and what he was just going to take in his stride. He didn't flinch when I talked about his high score on the Psychopath Test, but when I started talking about the possibility of a schizoid personality disorder, a disorder that is mostly about someone's disinterest in relationships and dislike of socialising, he became very agitated and we had to end the session. I can only imagine what it was like having Arthur live in your flat, with him malodorous, grumpy and frequently intoxicated.

Of course, this situation could not stand, and Arthur's new sister-in-law put her foot down: Arthur had to go. The couple confronted him together and offered to help him find a council place, but Arthur was absolutely incandescent about being forced out of a home he seemed to think he was entitled to live in, although he had absolutely no financial interest in it and contributed the bare minimum to the living environment. When he point-blank refused to leave, the argument became physical: a fight broke out between Arthur and his sister-in-law. Losing badly, Arthur ran to the kitchen and grabbed a kitchen knife, then made for his sister-in-law, whom he blamed entirely for trying to evict him and poisoning his brother against him. Then, as Arthur pulled back for a swing, he accidentally stabbed his brother in the thigh, nicking the femoral artery. Blood spurted out of the wound and his brother lost consciousness, and Arthur was literally a hair's breadth away from murdering his own kin. The ambulance crew arrived just in time to seal the wound and keep his brother from bleeding out. They were followed shortly by the police, and Arthur was jailed and charged with a Section 20 wounding. The judge who tried the case noted the existing charge for ABH and recent convictions for petty crime in addition to the wounding, and for whatever reason saw someone whose risk seemed to be escalating rapidly. He imposed the new sentence of indefinite imprisonment for public protection, meaning Arthur could spend his life in prison.

For most people, this would be a life-destroying moment, but in Arthur's case I sometimes wondered if it was, in fact, the best thing that had ever happened to him. Arthur seemed to flourish in prison: he needed a great deal of structure to keep him out of trouble and needed catering for. He loved repetitive activities and wanted to stay out of everyone's way as much as possible. Unlike most of the prisoners I worked with, I don't think Arthur was an addict as such; he used drugs and drank because that was what the people around him did when he was homeless. He just wasn't creative enough to think up another pastime so went along with it. In prison, he never seemed to particularly miss drugs or his life on the outside, and he sometimes seemed to find the idea of release terrifying.

Once, later on in Arthur's sentence, I set up a meeting to discuss a risk assessment with him relating to his plans following discharge. This was a bit hopeful given that he had an indefinite sentence but is standard practice; what I didn't know was how brutalising the whole experience was going to be for both of us.

It hadn't started well: there had been a miscommunication in the morning's timetable that had meant that Arthur had gone to the gym instead of his assessment meeting with me. Arthur loved the gym more than any other activity in prison and I knew he wasn't going to want to leave the session. However, Josie (who you may remember as the resolute psychologist from chapter two) had been absolutely clear that we were to notify the officers of any timetabling errors involving assessment sessions and have them corrected immediately. All the prison officers had a lot of respect for Josie, who had started out as an officer herself, so dropping her name tended to get things sorted out fairly quickly.

Arthur arrived ten minutes late for the session and understandably not in the best of moods, having been ripped away from his precious gym session to attend a meeting even I knew wasn't exactly the definition of urgency. When he walked in the room he was frowning so hard that the effect was like a villain from a child's cartoon when their secret plot has been foiled by a bungling hero. When combined with Arthur's regrettable tendency to keep a very narrow trimmed moustache with echoes of a German dictator, the overall effect was not of smouldering anger but camp comedy, which I doubt was his intention. He flopped into the chair opposite me and sulked. The officer accompanying him shrugged and nodded towards him as if to say, 'Sorry, guv, this isn't my fault.'

I sighed and opened my notepad.

'Hello, Arthur, thank you for coming here from the gym—'

'Yeah, well, I should be allowed to stay there, not fair to send someone to take me out once you've let me in there, is it? You're all the same, you lot, I—'

I interrupted. 'Now, Arthur: the regulations say that these sessions take priority over everything else. You have a copy of the timetable too and you can clearly see this is what you had in for this morning. Now, I wonder why you didn't let the officers know that the gym session was a mistake.'

(That wasn't really a question, I knew perfectly well why.)

'Hmph,' responded Arthur, also apparently aware this was not a question.

'So, we're here today to talk about the future section of your risk assessment. Like I said last week, this is all about plans you have made for after your release. Let's start with—'

'You WHAT?!' Arthur's eyes were wide open, his pupils dilated. He looked absolutely terrified.

'Plans you have made for ... after your release?' I ventured.

'I'm not fucking being released! Nobody told me about that, what the fuck do you mean?' His voice was about a full octave higher than usual.

'No, you're not being released, this is just about the fut—'

'You can't fucking release me! You don't have the right!' (He was definitely right on that count.)

'I'm sorry Arthur, I don't understand why you're upset. You're not going to be released soon, this is just forward-planning for when you are.'

But Arthur wasn't listening to me anymore. His 'head was gone': a prison expression for when an offender gets overcome with emotion and isn't thinking anymore, just following the anger.

'You can't fucking do this to me! I knew it, I never should have trusted you all here. You're all trying to get me sent away, away back to Belmarsh where they wouldn't even let me have gym. You're all working for *him*, aren't you?'

The officer was staring at Arthur wide-eyed. Like most staff, I don't think he'd ever seen Arthur do anything more emotional than drink a cup of tea, and it was taking him a while to process this almost Jekyll-and-Hyde-like transformation. He wasn't going to be much help if Arthur decided to go for me, so I decided I had to calm things down.

'Working for who, Arthur?'

'Prince Philip of course: you all are. All of you cunts!'

I thought better of pointing out that he was technically correct as this was Her Majesty's Prison Service. I dimly remembered that Arthur had a deeply held paranoid belief that Prince Philip had personally recommended he be sent to prison even though he had done nothing wrong. As far as he was concerned, at least.

'Look, Arthur, we just need to discuss this assessment. This isn't about whether you get released or not, it's just about what you plan to do when you're back in the community on your own.'

Every word of this was true, accurate and honest, and had Arthur's best interests in mind. It was also completely the wrong thing to say. Arthur got out of his chair, apparently with the intention of moving towards me, and at that moment the officer snapped out of his trance and his training kicked in. He sprang silently out of his chair and stood directly in front of Arthur, placing a large hand firmly on his shoulder.

'Come on now, Arthur, let's take a deep breath and sit back down, shall we?'

Arthur stared at him furiously for a second, then the realisation this was a fight he did not want to pick dawned and he complied, sullenly. Completely confused by how a conversation about release could have nearly ended in an incident,

I decided that we would end the session there. I asked the officer to take Arthur back to gym and figured Josie would be so interested to hear about Arthur's hidden emotional depths she wouldn't see this as a cop out.

I've no idea whether Arthur was standing up to gesticulate, shout more loudly or to attack me; I feel very fortunate that the officer was so experienced as to know when to intervene, and with just the right level of assertion, so that we never had to find out. Looking back, I think that Arthur was so terrified of any discussion about release from prison that he just wanted to shut it down. However, I also think that I'd inadvertently put myself in a situation where I was recreating the circumstances of Arthur's offence four years previously, which is never a good place to be.

Arthur's index offence, the reason he was in prison at the time, wasn't particularly unique in that the actual victim was not the original intended target of his anger, although that did add a tragic twist to his story. Rather, what was unique about Arthur was that, despite being a model prisoner in just about every respect, he was incapable of dealing with any complex emotion. He was at once absolutely dependent on the prison system and also completely unable to grasp that its purpose was not to provide him with a never-ending B&B stay with occasional waiter service (the prison was locked down once a month for training so staff would bring prisoners their meals to their cells), but rather to try to rehabilitate him.

I must confess that on this latter point we were rather lost. Working with Arthur over the next month, I could not find a single thing about life outside prison that would not be worse for him than the life he lived in prison: he was in every respect parasitic upon the prison system, just as he had been on his brother before and his mother before that. He was sad that his brother had been hurt but showed absolutely no remorse for attacking his sister-in-law, or empathy with their side of the situation that had led to the fight in the first place. Arthur also seemed to have changed the story of his offence around in his head so that it was the sister-in-law who had been holding the knife and stabbed his brother, contrary to the police report that had completely ruled out this version of events based on the location and angle of the stab wound.

After I had been working with Arthur for a couple of weeks, one of the prison physical education officers asked me if I would like to come along to the gym the next Friday. Arthur was going to be given an award, he said: apparently, he had completed a million miles on the 'ergo', the rowing machine. At the time, he was one of only five people to have achieved this feat (another prisoner, John MacAvoy, made news headlines in 2016 when he set a world record for the longest distance rowed on an ergo in 24 hours – 163 miles)[1]. I was dumbstruck: I had thought of Arthur as a parasitic psychopath who lacked the capacity for remorse, but what psychopath has the patience to put in enough hours to end up in an elite human endurance club? Psychopaths are supposed to be impulsive, explosive: they wouldn't have the patience to apply themselves to such a target and nor should they be able to go through the long learning process of pain, punishment and emotional reward.[2]

I thought about Arthur's case a lot, particularly about the incident with the risk assessment where he'd been unable to understand the idea of release being a hypothetical situation and thought I was trying to send him away from the prison. Over time, it occurred to me there might be another explanation for Arthur's behaviour. Poor socialisation, a very narrow range of interests, a literal mindset, inability to describe emotion, lack of empathy: these are all traits of high-functioning autistic spectrum disorder. The more time I spent with Arthur, and the more I read about this condition, I slowly became convinced that we had him all wrong; he was not a parasitic psychopath at all, rather he suffered from a disorder that was most likely genetic, and caused him to fundamentally lack interest in other people and socialisation. His lack of empathy made him pretty much the opposite of a psychopath: someone who was almost permanently at risk of being manipulated. A prison full of psychopaths was no place for such a vulnerable man. However, the only way to definitively diagnose someone with high-functioning autism is to interview someone who would have known him as a child, since this is when autistic behaviour is most prominent. Alternatively, we could find an expert in making these diagnoses in adults, but we were in a prison with only a team of mental health nurses to support prisoners' mental health.

Now as fate would have it, there was another prisoner on the wing who was behaving in a very rigid way. Derick (as he will be known) was engaged in a very odd, slightly perverse game with the prison officers where every morning, before he set off to work on the other side of the prison, he set up a row of chocolates in an apparently random order on the windowsill inside his cell. At that time there were concerns about prisoners getting access to mobile phones – BMW had just invented a phone that was about the size of a credit card, so room searches had increased in frequency, and of course the best time to search a prisoner's room is when they aren't there. So at least twice a week Derick would come back from his work to find that his chocolates had been moved from the meticulous arrangement he had placed them in, and he would not be happy. Initially this was probably just clumsiness on the behalf of the staff performing the search, who didn't realise how apparently critical the chocolates were to Derick's well-being; however, Derick started to bring this issue to the staff–prisoner business meetings that I had the pleasure of facilitating.

'I would just like to say that I have found that my possessions have been tampered with again,' Derick would say, voice faltering with high emotion.

To which another prisoner would reply, 'Fuck me ragged, not this shit again. Derick can't you just put the fucking things away.'

'No! These items are very important to me, they make me feel safe and secure in this madhouse. Why can't you understand that?'

One time, a senior officer, mustering every ounce of his considerable patience, said, 'Derick, we have made every effort to ensure that property is not disturbed in the searches. But this is a prison, and we don't determine the frequency of searches: that's set by the governor on the basis of,' the senior officer's eyes scanned the room, seeking out Paul, our old friend from chapter two, 'the presence of contraband in the prison.'

Paul's Machiavellian schemes were still very much on the down-low at this point and he was entertaining himself by provoking prison staff with the fact of his simple existence and an array of dismissive facial expressions. True to form, Paul smirked at the assembled staff and prisoners.

Immune to the senior officer's reasonable explanation, and perhaps inflamed by Paul's provocative expression, Derick became even more agitated.

'I don't understand why you need to search the windowsills. I mean, sweets aren't banned and a windowsill is very easy to see, and empty apart from my very specific pattern. WHY IS IT SO HARD FOR YOU TO JUST LEAVE THEM ALONE?' Emotion spread quickly around the room.

'I can't fucking believe I'm sitting in a room arguing about chocolates,' reflected another prisoner, previously silent in the meetings.

Then came the retort from another prisoner again. 'You can shut up, Staffy: we all know it's you who's been shitting in the showers every morning.'

'That's fucking it, come here you c—' and at that point Staffy and his interlocuter were helped out of the room by the prison officers. The meeting was abandoned. Derick seemed oddly pleased.

Now Derick probably comes across as very sincerely wronged in this exchange, and perhaps he was, but something about it didn't quite gel with me. Derick and Arthur were about the same age but that was about the only way they were alike: Derick was a regular at the horticulture group and often tried out other groups too 'for fun'. He loved engaging with the psychologists and got very bored and impatient whenever he had to give sustained attention to something. Worse still, there was something about the idea of arranging five very light sugary sweets, which the wind was probably as likely to disturb as a prison officer, that seemed to be asking for trouble, but with the absolute minimum of effort attached to it. I felt that this was a concerted attempt to provoke confrontation with the staff; one from which Derick would always come out looking like the wronged party. Nor could I understand how or why chocolates could have such emotional significance for anyone: where I'd seen obsessional 'hoarding' behaviour like this in the past, the hoarded objects had at least had some intrinsic value. A patient in a hospital I'd worked at before coming to the prison had hoarded pairs of Nike trainers; another had kept vintage fountain pens: all things where the value was clear. Chocolates were easily replaced, had no specific value and were, as Derick said, absolutely legal in the prison, meaning that – conveniently perhaps – there could be no resolution to the situation if the staff were to 'lose' the chocolates as Derick could just get more. For me, Derick was no Arthur, trapped in a world that was supposed to punish him. In fact, a lot of what I thought he was doing looked distinctly manipulative and perhaps even psychopathic.

My suspicion was that Derick was malingering, feigning his obsessive symptoms so that he had a righteous stick to beat the staff with and try to get transferred to a hospital, where he would have an easier time of it. However, one prisoner, especially Arthur, needing help was something that could be downplayed by the prison management, but if I could suggest that a psychiatrist also assess a menace like Derick, and perhaps arrange for him to be transferred alongside poor Arthur; well, that would be a result everyone could get behind.

Bringing the nurses onside with a heartfelt appeal on Arthur's behalf, we appealed to the governor about getting in an expert in autism to assess Derick and Arthur. A consultant psychiatrist and expert on autism was located and invited to the wing to review our men. Arthur could finally get the help he needed to find the life he never had and get out of prison, and Derick would be shown up as the shallow, psychopathic fraud he was and live out his jail time tormented by the chocolate removal group. That seemed to me like a just outcome.

It's rare that I get official documents from the Prison Service that I am enthusiastic about reading, and it was even rarer when I was in my late twenties. But on this occasion, I set aside time to read through the psychiatrist's report carefully, word for word. Derick's case was discussed first, and the psychiatrist had given a long narrative about his disturbed family life, inability to relate to other people and need for routine and ritual. In the conclusion, to my great surprise, he concluded that Derick was 'terribly ill-suited to a prison environment where his condition will only worsen' and 'must be transferred at the earliest convenience to my clinic where he can be given the specialist care he needs'. 'Huh,' I thought to myself. 'There's one born every minute.' Quickly though, my mind started to picture wing business meetings without a discussion of damnable chocolates, and I reasoned that I probably knew nothing about autism after all, and the psychiatrist expert probably had excellent judgement on such matters.

Then I read the section on Arthur, which I was a lot more invested in. It was meticulous, paraphrasing everything I had written in my assessment, including a beautiful section where the psychiatrist had measured the frequency of the nervous tic that Arthur developed when talking about his offending: 0.5 Hz, or one tic every two seconds. There was even a compliment on the thoroughness of my own assessment that made my cheeks prickle. However, it was the conclusion that really made my jaw drop. With it, the psychiatrist had fixed Arthur's fate: in his opinion, Arthur was a dangerous psychopath, who could not be helped by mental health services and should remain in prison for the rest of his sentence.

I couldn't have been more wrong.

I still have copies of these psychiatric reports and even with the benefit of over ten years of hindsight and multiple readings, I don't understand how the psychiatrist put together the same information into such a different picture to that which I had. For a long time, I thought that I must have been naive or ignorant in my understandings. Now, experience suggests that sometimes professionals working in mental health are just going to disagree about how they interpret what seem like solid facts. This is especially the case when they know that a lot is at stake in terms of protecting the public or controlling access to an expensive and precious resource like a forensic mental health clinic bed. However, I still get uncomfortable when I think about Arthur, on his rowing machine, totally dependent on the system for the rest of his life. The only consolation I have is that Arthur probably thinks this is all just fine, so long as interfering busybodies like me stay away from his case.

Chapter Six
Danny, The Borderline

It was my first day on the brand-new assessment ward at the hospital, in a specialised unit for men with severe personality disorder. I was being escorted by Jack, the modern matron who was also a veteran of some 30 years of psychiatric inpatient nursing. He was a sort of intimidating cross between Antonio Banderas and Yorkshire fast-bowler Freddie Trueman: good-looking but gruff and jaded, who said what he liked 'and liked what he bloody well said'. The ward was silent and a bit tense, as they tend to be when patients and staff are new and still trying to work things out, particularly how to avoid each other as effectively as possible. Jack was unfazed by this, presumably experiencing it every day, and being too large

141

a personality not to overcome any silence with bravado and banter.

We approached a young man, who can't have been much past 18 but had the pale, sallow complexion and red-raw eyes of someone who has already spent a lot of time in institutional care. He looked as though he might fall over from the breeze at any given moment, and it was at this moment that Jack adopted a boxer's stance and appeared to level a punch directly at the young man's head. For a split second all my paranoid fears reached a terrifying pitch, and I thought about how I would have to blow the whistle on a man and an institution I was just starting to developing some affection for; but the punch pulled up at the last moment and the young man collapsed in a fit of conspiratorial giggles. 'What's up, Jack?' he said to my companion. I wasn't sure who was the butt of the joke, if there was a joke.

This was my first introduction to Danny. Later that day I heard that he'd been left unsupervised in a medical examination room for a moment, giving him just enough time to insert a glass catheter into his penis and smash it in half. A colleague described him as 'a real heart-sink patient' and I wondered what this meant, although my heart was already breaking from this awful punishment he had chosen to inflict on himself.

In a sense, every patient who comes into a secure hospital is demoralising. They have usually had very rough lives, surrounded by varying degrees of neglect, abuse, criminality, drug abuse and mental illness, and over time this has ground them down to the point where they have committed a crime serious enough for a judge or jury to doubt the sanity of the person responsible. In other words, the crime will be serious, and the story will be traumatic and depressing in an existential kind of way. However, when we work with men and women who have been both victims and perpetrators of violence and abuse there are two things that particularly invoke feelings of despair; these are innocence and hope. When we see innocence in a serious offender, we also know that a huge chunk of that person's life and freedom has been lost over a moment of insanity. However, we also want to feel hope because it is far harder to give up on a young person in their early twenties than it is an 'old lag' in their late fifties serving out their fifth, sixth, tenth prison sentence. Put these two together and you have a heart-sink patient: you meet them and your heart sinks at their innocence; you read the case files about their offence and it sinks even further; and finally you watch them foil and sabotage every chance they have at rehabilitation, wasting all of their life away in institutions, and your heart is broken.

Danny came into the system young. His father had been highly abusive towards his mother and older brother before leaving the family for good when Danny was a small boy. His mother, who seemed like someone trying to make the absolute best of being dealt a terrible hand in life, had struggled with poor mental health, probably exacerbated by the physical abuse from her ex-husband and later partners. On a visit to the hospital, Danny's brother revealed that, when Danny was a baby, their mother had stored him in a drawer in the desk in the house to hide him from his father's wrath (although when Danny confronted her over this later she flatly denied it). When Danny was eight his mother was judged unable to care for him and Danny was taken into foster care.

Foster care is a difficult place for a young child, irrespective of the hardships they may have faced at home. Foster parents are very varied in their approaches to raising the children they take in, but the better ones will recognise their own limits and quickly return truly disruptive kids into social care. Danny had a safe initial placement but with a very large family, who had two of their own children and four other foster kids. Clearly the parents were very good at raising healthy children, but what they did not do was closely monitor what the kids got up to. Danny and his siblings would frequently go out around the town, searching for old buildings to play in, and sometimes steal or set fires. Once the kids, together with some friends, found a warehouse on the edge of town and went clambering around it. Danny was small and spry and found a way to climb up into the rafters of the building. Someone, Danny doesn't remember who, set a fire in the ground floor and the old, dry timbers quickly caught fire, trapping him upstairs. Fortunately, someone in the group noticed Danny was unaccounted for and called the fire brigade before legging it. The firefighters rescued him with nothing more than some minor smoke inhalation, but that was the end of his first relatively stable foster placement and he was taken into a care home. From that point on it was a chaotic series of foster placements, care homes and increasing involvement with gangs, who provided him a place to make some semi-stable friendships. Eventually he was discharged from the care system at 16 with some minor offences already on his police record, mainly low-level involvement in gang-related drug-dealing.

Trying to predict what this kind of diffuse, disrupted life will do to a young adult's personality is an alchemical art, but in Danny's case it played out with a kind of sick logic. Without a clear father figure, without his mother, and being passed around foster parents and the care system,

Danny never really had a chance to figure out who he was. Confused about how to be a man and angry with his missing mother for deserting him, even though she was virtually helpless (young men always seem to blame their mothers for the difficulties in their lives so they can remain strong like their awful, abusive fathers, identifying with the aggressors in their life),[1] Danny found the transition to adulthood extremely difficult. He tended to turn his rage and confusion inwards; harming himself with razors and knives and leaving terrifying scars – some of them on his face – that intimidated others and pushed them even further away. From what I could work out, even the gang leaders began to avoid him, presumably finding him too unstable and unpredictable for any serious work.

Identity confusion, emotional dysregulation, impulsive unpredictability and inwardly directed anger are often considered to be the core traits of a psychiatric condition called borderline personality disorder. Unlike psychopathy, it is formally recognised in the American Psychiatric Association's

DSM. Also unlike psychopathy, borderline personality is generally found to be more common in women than in men,[2] and there are many aspects of the disorder that seem incompatible with most of the key traits of psychopathic disorder. How can someone who does not care about others' perceptions of them be agonised by a lack of identity? How can a psychopath's callous unemotionality be compatible with emotional dysregulation? The short answer, of course, is that it can't, and the reason that someone like Danny can be a 'borderline psychopath' is more about the psychopath test, the PCL-R, than any real, separate disorder. Because more than half of the items in the test are about impulsivity and antisociality, some traits of psychopathy can coexist with borderline personality disorder to a high enough degree to give someone the diagnosis of 'psychopath', although they won't have some of the most core traits of the disorder. So, while the idea of a narcissistic borderline makes little sense, Danny's rage, fragility and absorption with his self-loathing did make him curiously dispassionate to, even callous about, the pain he inflicted on others.

Into this confused, angry young man's life came the Church of England, when a local vicar took a special interest in Danny. The church offered Danny some stability in a life otherwise dominated by chaos, and something approaching stability, rather like a gang. The vicar seemed unperturbed by Danny's extreme appearance, and they spoke regularly about faith and religion – even a life as a clergyman. I believe that Danny found something fundamentally important in these conversations: he sought to recreate this with many of the other religious leaders who worked at the hospital, deciding at various times to convert to Islam, Wicca and Satanism.

The fact that none of these stuck in hospital, however, might clue you in to the fact that it was in the community church that Danny's internalised chaos claimed its first serious victim. One of the most difficult and persistent problems of working with people with a diagnosis of borderline personality disorder is their hunger for identity, for something tangible to affix themselves to, so that they can look in the mirror and finally recognise themselves. As professionals, we often fall into the trap of trying to feed this bottomless hunger, of trying to 'fix' things; as if it is possible to find an identity on someone's behalf and fit it to them. In most cases we fail. We cannot fill the void, and instead of becoming heroes we are identified as failures and ultimately rejected. This rejection can take many forms, but perhaps there is something to the idea that the stronger the hunger, the more ferocious the response.

So it was with Danny: after some months attending church, helping out at events and having long discussions with the vicar, something was said that caused Danny to perceive a rejection. I have no way of knowing exactly what this was, as Danny didn't discuss his offence with anyone and the details in his case files were scant. However, from his interactions with the chaplain in the hospital, as they gamely and bravely tried to support his transitions between different belief systems, I came to understand the story.

Matters of faith and spirituality are necessarily loaded with emotion and feeling. Rejection from a faith is a terrible blow to the ego; likely why excommunication used to be considered such an awful punishment before the Enlightenment. My suspicion is that Danny wanted unconsciously to 'test' the vicar's commitment to him, to see if he was really another absent, untrustworthy father, and said something to try to provoke a rejection. Whether this was voicing curiosity about another religion, or – given Danny's taste for extreme actions and statements – possibly about Satanism, I don't know, but whatever it was, it was too much for the vicar and he angrily dismissed Danny. As the vicar turned to walk away, Danny produced a knife that he always carried with him and stabbed him in the back, puncturing a lung. Terrified of what he had done, Danny ran.

The vicar, although terribly injured, survived, called the police and Danny, who did not have either friends or trust from the criminal underworld to protect him, was quickly picked up and charged with attempted murder, later reduced to wounding with intent. This lesser offence still carries a potentially hefty sentence, and when Danny was convicted the judge took into account the nature of the attack – unprovoked, cold-blooded, attacking from behind – and sentenced him to ten years in prison.

Prison was not a good place for Danny, it is both boring and involves a lot of unsupervised alone time. He began to experiment with extreme ways of hurting himself, in particular searching for any means to emasculate himself, seemingly blaming his manhood for the terrible thing he had done. British prisons are tough places but prison staff know when they have met their match and applied for a hospital transfer, which meant that Danny would serve out his sentence in a secure hospital and would have to remain there until a psychiatrist deemed him safe enough to release. From the notes around his transfer, the psychiatrists assessing Danny had unusually few reservations about accepting him.

*

When I met Danny, the problem of self-harm was serious. He was not allowed anything that could be used to tie small ligatures as he would wrap these around his genitals to starve them of blood, so they'd drop off. As well as facial scarring, he had a persistent wound in his leg that he obsessively worried so it never fully healed, and that he could open up with a fingernail, producing large amounts of blood and pain virtually on demand. Most of the time his hospital room was an unusually sparse place as Danny proved able to turn the most mundane objects – compact discs, shoelaces, pens and pencils – against his body.

I found Danny easy to get on with at first, but the more time I spent with him the more difficult our interactions became. One period of seven days was particularly difficult: one Friday I was happily playing table football with him on the ward, by Wednesday my notes say that I found myself experiencing him as 'incredibly annoying' and as 'having a negative effect on my interactions with other staff and patients' – he insisted on following me around and telling me repetitively about his semi-delusional religious beliefs. The following Friday his mental state had become so unstable that he had been placed in seclusion by the nursing staff.

Having never seen a secluded patient prior to that point, I felt compelled – perhaps partly voyeuristically, partly out of a grim sense of scientific duty – to investigate. Danny was sitting naked on the bed, with no mattress (he had apparently found a way to remove the threads from the plastic to use as tourniquets around his penis) and his genitals firmly clenched between his legs – whether this was to hide his dignity or to attempt to disguise his own masculinity from himself or others was not clear. He heard me talking to the duty nurse observing him from the corridor and, smiling, tried to look for me, but I couldn't bring myself to meet his gaze or let him know I had seen him like this. Inside the seclusion area I saw a cold, alien image, like David Bowie in Nicolas Roeg's *The Man Who Fell to Earth*. The walls were covered with blood, and Danny had daubed a series of largely meaningless words together with a collection of what looked like pagan symbols in a pentagrammic shape. This blood had been taken from the wound on the inside of his leg. There were splashes of blood all over the floor and the bed, but nothing else in the room whatsoever but a steady flow of staff coming to look at the patient, almost as if this was a piece of extreme performance art. This felt voyeuristic and inappropriate, but the duty nurse justified it to me, saying that they were all involved in the patient's care and therefore needed to understand what they were dealing with better. As someone watching the watchers, I almost felt doubly guilty for being involved in this; I also hadn't been working in institutions long enough to have built a thick skin.

The scene had been harrowing and the incident left its mark. I had recurring nightmares about blood and alien environments for some weeks afterwards. My own interactions with Danny became very difficult following this experience, too; perhaps the hardest part being that Danny himself seemed completely unaffected by and dissociated from his behaviour that day: he wanted to talk to me as if nothing had happened, and I couldn't bring myself to reciprocate, to separate the man from the blood painter in his lonely cell.

In many ways I learned more from Danny than any other patient: his actions had reordered the way I thought about psychopaths and patients in general. He had reminded me that I had to find a way to limit the empathy I felt with them: not because they were undeserving of it, but because the potential damage to my own state of mind was too great. I wondered if this was why I was warned about heart-sink patients; it wasn't that they were dangerous to us physically, but rather to our own mental states. After working with Danny I was forced at once to create stronger boundaries about myself, and to approach my interactions with patients and prisoners in a much more clinical, and I worried also less authentic, way.

Danny's case showed me how paper-thin the line between psychopathy and insanity sometimes is. The distinction is a difficult and confusing one that comes very much from the unclear distinction between psychiatry and psychology. It is not helped by the fact that 'psychopathy' sounds similar to 'psychosis', which is a term referring to severe and usually acute forms of mental illness that impair someone's ability to understand reality; and it is nearly indistinguishable from 'psychopathology', which is a general term for any kind of disorder of the mind or brain. However, psychopathy is neither a mental illness nor a description of any kind of 'general' state of mind. Rather it refers to a condition that we believe is partly genetically based and partly about the kind of environment we encounter as we grow up, that results in some areas of the brain under-developing, usually those that control our ability to recognise emotions such as fear or sadness in others, and our ability to make effective calculations about risk.

This means that psychopaths are not like people with psychosis, who have 'too much' going on in their minds and lose contact with reality; nor are they suffering from a common or 'neurotic' kind of mental disorder such as depression or anxiety. Instead, they have failed to develop important parts of their personality, including the abilities to form lasting relationships or to show the warmth towards others that we all rely on to navigate us through life. There's a particularly resonant moment in series two of *Killing Eve* where narcissistic magnate Aaron Peel describes Villanelle as 'a void': it's an excellent characterisation because it draws attention to the idea that a psychopath is missing very important abilities that we all take for granted. Without them they have to function on 'best guesses' about people's reactions and how to mimic things like warmth and intimacy.

Danny hung on the most precarious of ledges between reality – albeit a warped kind of reality where emotions were always too hot, too intense and overpowering – and psychosis, a condition where he didn't seem to be in contact with himself at all, and this would let him do unspeakable things to himself and other people. Literally, he was almost constantly on this borderline, which is where the term comes from.

I'm almost done with Danny's story but there is something of an epilogue to it. When I was finishing up my time at the hospital, Danny had seemed much more stable and almost at peace. He had expressed to one of his psychologists that his quest to emasculate himself came from a place of wanting to change his gender as he was uncomfortable being a man. I thought this made sense: it explained where his disgust with his genitalia came from, and perhaps his dissatisfaction with his life choices so far. Better still, a medical doctor specialising in gender reassignment surgery had met with Danny and thought him an 'excellent candidate' for the surgery. On my last day, I found out that an appointment had been booked for a month's time where Danny would become a woman; a huge step for a young man and perhaps a braver one in the mid-noughties than it is today. All his clinical team were very supportive of the step.

Months later, I heard from a colleague that, just a week before the reassignment surgery, Danny had pulled out of the operation, saying he had been pushed into it by the consultant and it was all a 'misunderstanding'. I wasn't quite sure what to think about this: I had hoped that this surgery might have been the answer to Danny's problems, but I was wrong. I wondered how many more years of confusion he would suffer; whether he would ever find an identity he could stick with; and even if he did, whether this would be enough to get him released before he was no longer a young man.

Chapter Seven
Angela, The Remorseless

When I had my first placement at one of Britain's three high-security mental hospitals, at the age of 26, the personality disorder unit where I was based was a kind of 'hospital within a hospital', to get to which you had to walk all the way through the main hospital, along the corridor off which all the specialist wards branched, including the intellectual disability wards and the women's service. I had only been on the placement for about three weeks and was walking past the women's wards when the door slammed open, a good deal harder than anyone's blood pressure in a high-security hospital, especially mine, would ideally have liked. The group of people I was walking with immediately flattened against the wall (which had a thick padded section in

the middle) to maximise the thoroughfare and min-
imise our chances of being hit by flailing limbs. Out
through the door backed a nurse, moving jerkily as
if trying to catch a ball being thrown to him. He was
shortly followed by a large, nearly naked woman,
with smears of blood (her own? Another patient's?
Someone else's?) on her skin, screaming incompre-
hensibly and lashing out in virtually every direction,
with a clump of about six staff of all sexes, shapes,
sizes and grades (this was after the Blom-Cooper
report of 1992[1] so nobody wore uniforms), desper-
ately trying to get a hold of her. The flailing limbs
and screeching noises made the restraint scenes in
Nicolas Winding Refn's *Bronson* look like a Tom and
Jerry caper: this was a matter of life and death.

'Shower time,' muttered one of the nurses gno-
mically as the clump, having got a firm grip on the
still-screaming, still-struggling and still-bloody
woman, marched past us towards the recreation
area in the centre of the hospital. I wasn't sure if
this was an explanation or a destination.

I turned to give my best 'What the fuck?' glance
to the person next to me: it was Johnny, a recently

qualified clinical psychologist who I had met on induction a few weeks before.

'That's going to be my ward,' he said, in a voice that made me think of a British Tommy about to go over the top.

I was shocked at what I had witnessed. Over time I came to think that prisons and secure hospitals are structured and operated in a way that seems to torment and antagonise female patients in the same way as it provides an odd kind of containment for men like Arthur. Where men become aggressive and 'difficult' when they find institutions hard to cope with, this closed existence seems to cause female prisoners and patients to attack themselves; to injure and destroy their own bodies.[2] I have always found this much harder to deal with emotionally than the consequences of interpersonal violence; I think because with a case of 'typical' physical violence the divide between victim and perpetrator is clear, but with self-harm the patient is at once perpetrator and victim, and it can be very difficult to reconcile your anger at the perpetrator part with your empathy with the victim part.

Perhaps the fact that women struggle to cope with incarceration isn't too surprising. Prisons and asylums are institutions designed by men, for men, and can seem dehumanising enough even towards men. No thought has been paid to women's places in them, and it wasn't until 2007 that the UK health service started to develop services like The Orchard Unit in Southall that are designed specifically for the needs of female offenders with a mental disorder, not an afterthought tacked onto a male prison or hospital.

The idea of a female psychopath seems to capture the imagination of writers and artists in a unique way. If the government estimated that there were only 40 female criminal psychopaths in 2002 and 2,000 male, then the literature looks a little skewed. The portrayal of Aileen Wuornos in *Monster*, *Killing Eve's* Villanelle or *Dangerous Liaisons'* Marquise de Merteuil are all enduring characters, with countless parallels in less well-known films, books and TV shows: the female psychopath exists more concretely in our media than she does in reality. As

I said in chapter one, we know so very little about real female psychopaths that it seems somewhat bizarre that so many writers should decide to take them on as characters.

There seem to be two ways to write a female psychopath in fiction. The most common approach is to keep the same emotional and interpersonal features of psychopathy that are present in men, but subtract the 'messy' antisocial and lifestyle aspects (impulsivity, parasitism, general criminality) and replace them with a propensity to seek control of others through seduction and manipulation. The other approach, which I think is harder to nail because it goes against the grain of what we think women are, is to just write a woman as you would a male psychopath – a messy, brutal, remorseless criminal – and see how far you can get away with it. When Phoebe Waller-Bridge said that she'd used a murderer from Arizona USA, Angela Simpson, as part inspiration for the character of Villanelle, I was intrigued. The rarity of female psychopaths is one of the reasons I don't have much experience of working with them; but, frankly, the second reason is that I find them terrifying, much more so than men. Often that which we fear most also intrigues us, and so here I am.

I can see why Angela Simpson is a good case for an examination of a real-life female psychopath. Her crime was needlessly brutal and relentless, and for a while she gave a vast number of TV interviews where she almost seems to revel in unveiling her callous lack of empathy and remorse for her crime to reporters. In many ways she comes across as a monster: the kind of killer that serial-killer obsessives would have collected books over had she not been caught so early in her spree.

Angela Simpson was already acquainted with a 46-year-old man named Terry Neely, a former convict who appeared to have taken a shine to her, perhaps a sexual attraction or perhaps, as one documentary speculated, because she was a strong woman who had strong negative beliefs about the police and their persecution of minorities[3]. Apparently to impress Simpson, Neely told her that while in prison he had snitched on a man he shared a cell with, and implied (seemingly without any basis) that he was also an informant for the police. This was the wrong thing to say, however, as Simpson had decided that snitches were absolutely at the top of her hitlist, even ahead of sex offenders and the police.

Some days later, in August 2009, Neely ran into Simpson again, and she offered him drugs and sex if he came back to her apartment. Neely, a wheelchair user, complied, and Simpson persuaded him to leave his wheelchair outside the apartment, which as we shall see becomes significant later. Upon entering, though, he was tied to a chair in front of a mirror and then subjected to a horrifying two days of torture. Simpson repeatedly beat him unconscious with a tyre iron and stabbed him over 50 times with a variety of knives. She then extracted his teeth with pliers, and drove a three-inch nail into his skull using a hammer. Waking up the next morning, Simpson finally killed Neely by strangling him with a TV cable and then dismembered his body. She called her accomplice – a skinhead named Edward McFarland – and the two of them borrowed a neighbour's van to dump Neely's remains in a garbage can outside a local church and set fire to it. Apparently, Simpson actually told the van owner – who was later called as a witness – that she had killed Neely and needed the van to dispose of the body.

Because this case is so much in the public domain, and because of the very 'classical' way she presents as a psychopath, there are a few things about Angela's case that illustrate some very important points about psychopathy and human development. The questions I am really trying to answer here are: what makes a psychopath? And, what might be different about a real female psychopath?

Simpson's crime is not a particularly complex one, although it is on the more brutal side of killings as far as my experience goes. What is more complex is Simpson's forensic and developmental history: the details are sketchy and Simpson herself tells multiple, contradictory stories to different interviewers about her history, motivations, details about her offence and even the number of her victims.

What we do know is that Simpson was born in 1975 in Phoenix, Arizona. Her childhood has been reported as being 'chaotic', and she was repeatedly placed into foster care as a result of physical and sexual abuse within the family as a child;[4] Simpson describes being 'hospitalised' from the age of ten for psychiatric issues. Perhaps as a result, she developed a drug habit[5] in her early adulthood. She had four children before her early thirties, but considering her drug problems, a court determined that they should live with their grandmother. To fund her drug addiction, Simpson turned to sex work, and as far as we know this was her primary source of income.

Why Simpson suddenly decided to turn from a drug-using sex worker, someone who was likely victimised by drug-dealers and abusive clients, into a self-righteous 'avenging angel' is not clear. What we do know is that in June 2009, aged 33, she looked up a known sex offender in the area and, together with Edward McFarland, broke into the man's house, tied him up, beat him and robbed his property, warning him that they would be back.

The police did not initially connect Simpson to the crime.

In August 2009, three days after Neely last left his house, the local pastor was 'awakened to the smell of burning flesh' outside his church. The fire brigade were called, and when they found human remains they notified the police. Although they could identify the victim, the police could find no evidence of who might have done this to him, and nor could they find Neely's wheelchair.

Shortly after this, Simpson was arrested and jailed for an armed robbery she had committed two months earlier, where she had tied up the victim – a convicted sex offender – and threatened him repeatedly. Figuring that the modus operandi in the two cases was similar and having spoken to the neighbour who had lent Simpson the van, the police checked Simpson's apartment. Sure enough, the missing wheelchair was outside, and inside they found enough evidence of Neely's blood to be sure that they had their killer. They charged Simpson with murder in the first degree (the most serious murder charge in the USA) and McFarland with aiding and abetting. Simpson 'proudly' confessed to killing Neely to the police in interview but pled not guilty in court, presumably to avoid the death penalty.

In the months between Simpson's arrest and her court case, she gave several interviews to local reporters, who visited her jail, where she suggested that she did commit the crime and that she was glad she did it. I can't imagine her defence attorney's face on seeing some of this footage on national television as one of the primary conditions of the charge is that the killing is both 'wilful' and 'premeditated', arguably both things that Simpson strongly evidenced in her appearances. It's these interviews that I think became the main basis of Simpson's celebrity, and the material that Phoebe Waller-Bridge described as 'gold dust' when looking for inspiration as to how to characterise Villanelle.

One of the most revealing pieces of footage relating to the case is a short section from an interview Simpson gave to a 3TV reporter in 2012

– it's the most popular hit for her name on Google. Right towards the start of the interview, the reporter asks, 'Why did this man deserve to die? You claimed he was a snitch, but ...'

Simpson responds immediately, almost interrupting: 'Well, he told me he was a snitch, on many occasions, but that doesn't matter. Why did you guys want to kill me?'

'What?'

'[The city of] Phoenix wanted to kill me. What's the difference? Everybody has a reason to kill. My reason might not be good to you, but your reason wasn't any good to me.'

'Umm ...' stumbles the reporter.

Although he is pursuing a deeply stupid line of questioning – asking a psychopath for moral reasoning about her victim – Simpson pounds the reporter's argument into dust through a ferocious pseudo-logic that plays on the moral equivalence of murder and capital punishment. Surely the reporter is there to interview a murderer who has already shown her absolute lack of remorse in previous appearances: why go digging here? Is he surprised to find a woman who effectively stares him down like a man would, rather than give him 'soft' answers that might placate the audience and make her appear more sympathetic? When the reporter continues with a prurient line of questioning about the offence ('What exactly happened over those three days?'), he gets a withering stare and, 'What do you mean?' Simpson is mocking him, pushing the interviewer to describe the crime when it clearly makes him uncomfortable. However, in this respect Angela reminds me a lot of Paul: they both seem to want, consciously or otherwise, to see people squirm as they assume as much control as they can in the interview.

There are a few aspects of Simpson herself, if not her case, that I think are particularly interesting. For a variety of reasons, I think there is a high probability that Simpson is a psychopath. First, the court ordered two psychiatric evaluations during her pre-trial hearings: had they found any evidence of severe mental illness, such as schizophrenia, she would have been referred to a specialist mental health court, but this did not happen. Psychopathy, as it is not listed as a mental disorder in the main diagnostic systems (although its common partner antisocial personality disorder is), is not usually recognised as a basis for an insanity defence, so the most likely outcome of the psych evaluation was either no disorder or psychopathy.

Second, Simpson has most of the features of primary psychopathy: she has no remorse for her crime and has a callous and unemotional attitude towards her victim; she is glib and superficial in her interviews, citing a poorly defined criminal code as the explanation for her offending ('snitches get stitches') when she has no extended criminal record that suggests she knows about policing or prison; she feels she is in some way 'entitled' to take life, which displays considerable grandiosity in her worldview; and she is clearly given to anti-social behaviour, breaking rules, taking illegal drugs and being sexually promiscuous.

Notably lacking in this list is any indication that she shares the characteristics of the most common fictitious female psychopaths I noted at the start of the chapter: she isn't particularly given to conning or manipulative behaviour. McFarland, who helped her dispose of the body, quickly turned against her in court, suggesting no allegiance to, or belief in, Simpson and her crusade. In her interviews she made little attempt to charm and seemed to have little time for presenting herself in a positive light. She arguably manipulated Neely into coming to her apartment, but perhaps it would not be a difficult task to attract a loner with mobility issues and a criminal history into the flat of a woman known to engage in sex work.

What is most interesting, though, is how the perception of Simpson as a psychopath relates to what we perceive as 'male' and 'female' characteristics in society and how these translate into our mythology and cultural understandings of psychopathy and killers in general. The way Simpson acts challenges the idea of the 'feminine' psychopath: rather, she presents herself in the same way as a male psychopath does. There are, for example, clear similarities with Ted Bundy's notorious 'confession' videos from the late 1980s. Extensive and intense eye contact, an evident disinterest in emotionally engaging with the reporter's highly charged questions. Both Simpson and Bundy also have a simple, clear defence or rationalisation for what they have done: Simpson thinks informants need to die and views her conviction as an unfortunate but unavoidable consequence of her righteous crusade; Bundy views himself as a victim of pornography use and sees this as a 'plague' affecting young men in the USA. In both cases, two people in prison for life, Bundy awaiting his imminent execution, wrestle absolute control of the interview away from their interlocutor: they dictate their appearance in the eyes of the viewer, they use the interview to advance their view of the world and they never get emotional or distracted by the line of questioning or obvious appeals to emotion. The reporter asked Simpson about her children and she responded, simply, 'I don't want to talk about my children.'

In short, Angela Simpson presents with virtually the same spread of traits as a male psychopath: she is not a 'gendered' psychopath. Nor can it be

coincidence that Aileen Wuornos, the female killer probably most associated with psychopathy
in women, presents in much the same way: an
aggressive predator without conscience,[6] not a
manipulator of others. Some research studies
have found some differential patterns in the
presentation of male and female psychopaths,
where women are more deceitful and less antisocial overall,[7] but these also don't match up
with the literary or popular stereotypes of the
femme fatale. Both Wuornos and Simpson used
their sexuality to some extent in their offending, but sexuality – or rather, the use of sexual
desire and intimacy to control and manipulate
– was central to Paul's case, as it was to Ted
Bundy's.

In the interview for 3TV, Simpson is invited to
dwell on the idea of whether her gender affects the
way she is perceived. The interviewer asks:

'You're sort of an interesting character because,
first of all … women don't commit crimes this
heinous.'

'Right.'

'Usually this kind of crime is more the domain of men.'

[Smiling] 'That's unfortunate.'

'You think more women should … ?'

'Oh yeah, equal opportunities, definitely.' [Smirks]

Simpson is playing with the interviewer here, of course, but the 'equal opportunities' comment is interesting. She seems to be saying that these kind of stereotypes about women as incapable of remorseless, psychopathic crimes are invalid, almost as though she is making a case for more female serial killers. It's very likely that this is why Phoebe Waller-Bridge drew on these interviews in fleshing out the character of Villanelle in the *Killing Eve* series: to ask the question 'what would a female psychopath be like if they were thrown into a male role'. I think this juxtaposition is so powerful because it reminds us exactly how we expect women to behave onscreen: to be weak or contrite when they are violent, or to be a cynical 'manipulator' psychopath, like the Marquise de Merteuil, rather than an enforcer like Villanelle or any number of male hit-man characters. Villanelle gets a licence for callous, remorseless, even evil behaviour that we accept and even applaud in male psychopaths such as Dexter, but one we haven't seen before in female characters.

There is another interesting question here about what a psychopath is 'supposed' to be in society's eyes. Simpson's case seems to inspire, more than any of the other stories in this book, use of the word 'evil' to describe her and her actions. Of course, the liberal use of this term may have something to do with the fact that she was a black woman from a poor neighbourhood, whereas Jason Marshall, who was also 'almost' a serial killer, is often depicted as confused and failed by the system. But can anyone be inherently 'evil' and what would this mean?

The idea of 'evil' is a major contributor to some of the more draconian ideas about how psychopaths are managed in criminal justice systems across the world, from near-permanent isolation in the US supermax system to the indefinite confinement of the 'long-stay' programme in the Netherlands, where there is no maximum sentence and offenders can remain in custody for the rest of their lives. It's also wrong-headed as it confuses 'amorality' – that is, being without a moral compass in the way a psychopath is – with 'immorality', or being fundamentally wicked. Sure, it may be true that there are 'evil' people in the world, and it may be that some of them are psychopaths; however it is not the case that all psychopaths are 'evil', or even that they have learned very basic distinctions between 'good' and 'bad' that you and I take for granted. This is in part because their brains are not wired to learn in a similar way to a non-psychopath:[8] they are focused on satisfying their basic needs and whichever primitive (in the sense of almost child-like) desires they have developed during their infancy.

When considering Angela Simpson's case, my impression is that, feeling a failure as a mother and a provider, she was driven to find something within her life that she could view as 'good'. By terrorising and taking the lives of men she then believed to be evil, who contributed to the bad things in her life by

committing sexual abuse or informing on 'good' criminals, she found a way to show herself that she was
not a bad person. I think she probably saw herself
as the opposite of a bad person: a kind of avenging
angel. Perhaps this audacity – in a woman, of all
things – was why the judge chose to sentence her to
natural life in prison, plus an additional 14 years: a
unicorn sentence for a unicorn offender.

About six minutes into Simpson's famous 3TV
interview, the reporter asks an interesting question, or at least one that has bothered me somewhat
about the case given the police's flat denial of any
involvement with her victim. He asks:

'That's what did it [for] him ... the bragging
about putting people in prison, people you knew?'

Simpson responds, 'No, I didn't know any of
them, no.'

'Do you believe him? Do you think he was a
snitch?'

'Well ... "oops" if he wasn't!'

Chapter Eight
Eddie, The Redeemed

It doesn't get much further away from the stereotypes than this. I've come to meet a psychopath, not in the safety of a hospital or a prison surrounded by burly guards, but in a house in a very normal north London street. Two small dogs caper around our feet while we drink very decent espresso from Eddie's espresso machine and eat cakes. Eddie tells stories, I tell stories: we laugh. We have an in-joke about why he is called 'Sid'. Eddie tells me about his past, about growing up in a dysfunctional and sometimes abusive family; about the people who have died because of his actions. I try to listen and be perceptive but fair in my questions. Sometimes I think Eddie perceives me to be a bit of a 'right one'; sometimes, despite my best efforts, I think I am judging him for what he did many years ago. Still, it feels we both have a job to do here, and that is to understand how Eddie went from taking someone's life when in his twenties and spending time in a secure mental hospital to sipping espresso in domestic bliss. It's a complex story, full of anger, despair and violence, but also in many ways the most powerful case in the book.

Working in services for severe personality disorder, it's an unfortunate fact of life that you will get used to having your heart broken by your clients, just as Danny did to me when I was very new to it all. A few years after working with him I did a very short piece of work with a charity that catered for men and women with severe psychotic disorders, such as schizophrenia. I was only there for a couple of weeks, but after I left I got a couple of lovely letters from clients thanking me for giving up my time to help them. I was absolutely taken aback: in 15 years of work with personality-disordered offenders I have never had a single letter of thanks. It's entirely possible I'm a dreadful person and an inept clinician, but I also think that, in the eyes of the people I've worked with who have become success stories, I am the last thing they want to think of.

Perhaps more importantly, though, I've seen how the system and the clients can fail each other terribly: men I've worked with have been sent back to prison because they aren't willing to change anything about themselves in therapy; others who make it all the way to the hospital gate (literally) only to sabotage their progress with a stupid decision and remain inside for another year or more. I've also worked with men who progressed through the system and were successfully discharged, but then re-entered the system, usually by breaching the terms of their release, only for me to meet them again going the wrong way into more secure care as I moved down from high-security to medium-security work. Heart-sink, indeed.

I have been aware of Eddie's case for a long time, and we met once in person at a conference a few years back, but I'd never spent much time with him before today. I decided to approach him about being interviewed for this book because his former doctor, a brilliant forensic psychotherapist who supervised me for five years, always viewed Eddie as one of her greatest success stories. Eddie, she would say, just seemed to get the idea that changing yourself was not something anyone else could do for you: you had to take responsibility for what you had done and for the process of change before you could even begin. This sounds so easy, but it was this very step that over half of the men I worked with never seemed to 'get': they always wanted to blame someone else for them ending up in prison or a secure hospital. Now Eddie isn't the only man I know to set his life straight, but he certainly had the highest hill to climb in order to achieve this, because when he was a younger man he did some terrible, scary things.

Eddie is quite an intimidating presence, even though he's in his fifties now and sometimes uses a cane to get around. He is a big man: tall and well-built, and his hands seem enormous, like a northern warrior from *Game of Thrones*. He is polite, and extremely generous to me both with his time and his energy, but he has a directness to his speech and movement that makes you wonder what it's like to get on the wrong side of him. Sometimes he talks about feeling his temper rise when someone behaves badly in a queue on the street, but Eddie has made his mind up that losing control of his emotions is just not something that interests him anymore: he has moved on.

The story he has to tell of how he got to this place is a very instructive one, because it helps us to understand what can go so badly wrong in someone's life for them to end up being called a psychopath.

Eddie was born near the Docklands area of London in the 1960s. This wasn't a good time for the London docks: following the Blitz, when they were almost completely destroyed, they had a golden period of rebuilding and success, but eventually they were unable to support the massive container ships that now dominate international naval trade. As a result, between 1960 and 1981 the docks were slowly demobilised and demolished, leaving behind local communities who had relied on them for jobs, social investment and economic development.

Eddie's childhood and young adulthood was intimately connected to the docks, both through the work that went on there and the less salubrious aspects of dock life, including illegal goods, drugs, smuggling and other petty crime. His biological father died when Eddie was very young, and his mother started another relationship soon after, which produced a younger half-brother, Charlie, to go with Eddie and his older brother Dan. Life around this time sounds fairly normal for Eddie and his brothers: his stepfather, Martin, was a bit of a wheeler-dealer and a ladies' man, but both parents were in work and the kids were minded by their maternal grandmother. From the age of six or seven, Eddie described doing things with his friends and brothers that we might describe as 'rascally' – playing 'Knock down Ginger' (knocking on a house door and running away); sneaking a £20 note from Martin's wallet and going on spending sprees in London, leaving his mother to take the rap; stealing goodies like cream, cheese and yoghurt from the milk float when the milkman stopped to make deliveries in a high-rise block. Sometimes he'd get shouted at by his stepfather, but his behaviour was nothing very unusual.

Things started to go awry for Eddie when he was ten. Sick of Martin's womanising, Eddie's mum left him and found a new boyfriend. Initially charming to the whole family, once he had 'got his feet under the table', as Eddie put it, he started to become far more domineering with his wife and stepchildren, physically abusing them and enforcing a tyrannical system of discipline that meant he was completely in control of family life. Eddie describes him being like a 'sergeant major', constantly shouting and giving disciplinary beatings.

One time, Eddie came up the stairs in the house to find his new stepfather dragging his mother into the bedroom by the hair, something that upset him enough to pick up a knife from downstairs and come back to 'do him'. When he went into the bedroom, however, he saw them having sex, which confused and disgusted him. He was unsure whether this meant that everything was OK, but with the hindsight of an adult he is certain that his stepfather was raping his mother. He said that he always lived with the guilt of not doing anything, but at the same time felt betrayed that his mother allowed it to happen, even though she was probably just trying to survive.

Eddie's stepfather started to play mind games with the boys: Eddie recalled a particularly unnerving episode when he was 13 where he woke up in the morning to find that the room he shared with Charlie was on fire. As he told me the story:

'The fire was all over the place, little fires here and there. My hands were all burned up and swollen from trying to get out of the room. All of a sudden, my stepfather comes running up the stairs, trying to get us out, like, "Come on, come on!" My little brother was blamed for starting the fire, but he was only four or five at the time and I truly believe in my heart that it was my mother's husband – *that fucking thing* – who did it, just so he could be the hero.'

I asked Eddie whether he thought that his stepfather intended to hurt them: he said no, but we kicked it around for a while, and Eddie said he thought perhaps this was a way of playing 'cuckoo' with his wife's children: by setting a fire and ensuring the children would be blamed, he then had the ability to get the kids sent away so he could monopolise their mother. Whether this is true or not, that was exactly what happened: Dan was sent to his aunt's house and Eddie and Charlie were sent to live with Martin, where he stayed for a couple of years. Now 15, Eddie had decided to leave school, and Martin gave him a job working for his construction company. However, he was paid only £8 a day, less than a third the wage of the older workers, who made £25, which made Eddie feel exploited. Eddie's behaviour began to worsen during this period – hardly surprising as his family was being broken apart – and he started to hang out with older boys, stealing cars and pinching goods from the containers in the docks that were often left unattended.

One day Eddie simply refused to go to work, with what sounds like steadfast teenage obstinacy. Martin's new wife shot him a look of contempt, and in response Eddie picked up the keys to Martin's car and drove off down the road. The police eventually caught up with him, so Eddie ditched the car in a supermarket car park and hid between two freezer units. However, in what was to become something of a recurring theme in Eddie's criminal life, there was a stroke of serious misfortune: an off-duty senior policeman happened to be doing his shopping, caught sight of him and directed the uniformed bobbies to Eddie's hiding place. He was taken to the police station and the arresting officers found a gold bracelet, without any packing or receipt, in the glove compartment. The bracelet actually belonged to Martin, and although it was not completely legal – as no tax had been paid on it – it was not stolen. However the police assumed it was, and worked Eddie over about where it had been nicked from – Eddie observed drily that the story concocted by the arresting officer, where Eddie's non-existent girlfriend, who worked in a non-existent jewellery shop, was handing him stolen gold bracelets to fence, would make a 'decent book, maybe better than yours, Mark' – but after getting nothing out of him the police went to arrest Martin and put him in the cell next to Eddie.

Eventually one of them made a phone call to Eddie's uncle, who actually was a gold dealer, and he managed to concoct a plausible enough story to get both of them released. However, although Martin did not press charges over the car, he was not pleased with Eddie: 'I'm too old for this shit: you'll have to go back to your mum's.'

Back with his mum, Eddie went back to school briefly, but he was very affected by the break-up of his family and continued to engage in what he calls 'skullduggery': hanging out at the docks, causing trouble, breaking into cars and occasionally fencing stolen goods in a local pub that seemed to be a hive of black market sales. He had also started seeing a woman in her early twenties called Mary, who lived near the docks and who, according to Eddie, had a reputation for 'entertaining' schoolboys in their late teens with sex and drugs. Eddie met Mary after making a prurient trip to her place with a friend, which from the way he put it sounds like something of a rite of passage for Docklands boys, but their relationship became closer than most.

This all changed quickly, however. One lunchtime Eddie and a group of six kids from his school went over to the comprehensive next door and started causing mischief, tipping tables and drawing on the walls. As soon as a teacher from the comp spotted them, they ran back to their own school, but the teacher followed them. The boys were made to do a line-up, and the teacher pointed out just Eddie as one of the trespassers: again, unlucky as he was one of the six trespassers. This was the 1970s, so it is possible that Eddie might have faced a caning for this (corporal punishment was outlawed in the UK in 1986), but Eddie told me that wasn't the reason for what happened next. Perhaps reminded of his abusive stepfather waggling his finger, Eddie lost his temper, 'went a bit psycho' as he put it, and attacked the teacher, punching him and punching him, until two of his own teachers pulled him off. The teacher was unharmed; he seemed to know how to defend himself (perhaps this was a necessary qualification for working in an east London school at that time), but the police were called and arrested Eddie again. He was suspended from school and charged with actual bodily harm.

Eddie was sentenced to three months in a detention centre (what would now be a young offenders' institution), which was difficult: he felt bullied by the staff, although no more than anyone else – 'they were shitbags to everyone and we were treated like dogs', Eddie put it punchily – and got into several fights with the other inmates. However, he did make one friend, and they happened to be released on the same day.

On the day of his release, Eddie's mother made the train journey across the country to collect him. It was quite cold, so she had brought along his favourite coat, something he now recognises as a lovely gesture. At the time, however, he was embarrassed to be seen to be a 'mummy's boy' in front of his friend. After they made the journey back to London, rather than coming home with his mother, Eddie left her at the station and went straight to see Mary, the older woman by the dock-side, leaving his mother distraught. 'I was just thinking with my other fella,' he put it.

He started smoking cannabis with Mary and taking diethylpropion, a weight-loss tablet similar to amphetamines that she had a regular supply of from the dockworkers. 'I knew she was very pro-miscuous, but I was very needy ... I needed to be attached to someone,' Eddie told me. 'I don't know if I maybe needed a family because mine was split up; there was a lot of confusion in my mind. I became infatuated with her and extremely jeal-ous and extremely insecure: I was controlling, but I expected her to be faithful to me while I was out with other ladies. I was always terrible to her: I'd slap and punch and kick her, it was horrendous.' Eddie also started to take more to drinking, hang-ing out in the pub with his friends. Despite only being 15 or 16 at the time, the landlords took little notice: 'We were cash-paying customers and could probably pass for 18 most of the time.'

If this sounds like a volatile situation – drugs, alcohol, jealousy, infidelity, domestic abuse – then it certainly ended dramatically, with Mary holding a large knife to Eddie during an argument in the kitchen. 'Go on then, stick it in me,' he remembered mocking her, not believing she would do it, but Eddie had miscalculated the seriousness of the situation, or perhaps Mary's instability, and she stabbed him in the abdomen. He had to be rushed to hospital for stitches, and although there was no lasting damage, that was the end of Eddie's first real relationship with a woman.

Often psychologists talk in quite general terms about 'adverse childhood experiences' (ACEs) that can have consequences on a child's emotional and intellectual development as well as increasing their chances of being both victims and perpetrators of violent crime.[1] In Eddie's case, we have the detail we need to understand the impact of the abusive, controlling behaviour his family suffered at the hands of his second stepfather. Murderously angry with his stepfather for abusing him and his brothers, and sexually dominating his mother, Eddie came to look for signs of this behaviour in all the male authority figures he met, from Martin to the schoolteacher, while at the same time blaming his mother for bringing the abuser into his home and submitting to him. If this logic sounds flawed – after all, how could Eddie's mum have defended herself, let alone her sons, from a larger, aggressive man – this may be because of a psychological process called 'identification with the aggressor' that I identified with Danny in chapter six. Eddie did not want to see himself as abused, and therefore weak by the standards of masculinity at the time, so despite hating him he came to act more like his stepfather – violent and controlling in relationships – and saw his mother as weak and culpable. He unconsciously edited out emotions and memories that suggested she was not complicit but helpless: being controlled, raped and beaten by her partner. In Eddie's mind this was how women had to be: weak victims who were complicit in every beating they received.

His first relationship and heartbreak behind him, Eddie was back at his mum's house, still smoking cannabis and financing his habit by stealing from containers being stored at the docks. It wasn't long before he met another girl, Jeanne, and began another very intense relationship with her. After about nine months, when they were both 17, they discovered Jeanne was pregnant. Eddie's docks income wasn't stable or high, and he needed money to finance a family. His first port of call was to go back to Martin, who really seemed to have a soft spot for Eddie. He asked him, 'Can you get out of bed in the morning?' and when Eddie promised him 'yes' Martin offered to take him back on, forgiving the theft of his car. When Eddie asked about the pay, however, Martin's response was '£8 a day', the same rate he had always paid him and still a third of the rate of the older workers. Eddie took this extremely personally, as if he wasn't worth any more in Martin's eyes than he was two years ago. As he described it to me, Eddie 'lost the plot', punching Martin in the jaw and storming out. Perhaps to teach Eddie a lesson, Martin thought that it was a good idea to press civil charges against him, but he insisted on conducting his own prosecution, which rather backfired. When the judge asked Eddie why he'd hit the plaintiff, Eddie responded:

'Well he was only paying me eight pounds an hour.'

'That's a reasonable rate for someone his age, your honour,' responded Martin.

The judge nodded approval and looked at Eddie. Eddie searched his head for something to say.

'Yeah, well ... what about the tax?' he said. 'The tax you're meant to pay on the other guys?'

The judge looked at Martin, cocking his head. What about the tax, indeed?

Martin went rather pale and silent. The judge frowned.

'Case dismissed,' he said.

With the child's birth coming ever closer, Eddie became desperate: with Jeanne he planned a confidence heist on a local jewellers. Eddie would walk in and ask to see some bracelets, then Jeanne would come in off the street and open the door long enough for Eddie to pick up the tray of bracelets and run out with them, making it appear like an opportunistic theft with no involvement from Jeanne. Unfortunately, this was not something out of *Ocean's Eleven*: a woman overheard what the two of them were planning outside the shop and secretly notified the staff. When Jeanne came in, the staff locked the door after her and called the police, who arrested both of them. Eddie pleaded guilty, which meant the police didn't press charges against Jeanne, but also meant that Eddie went back to prison, this time to borstal – a kind of detention centre with an emphasis on training and rehabilitation.

Eddie says he didn't mind the borstal so much, although he bullied the other inmates and kept getting involved in fights, but he remembers how he became obsessed with phoning his girlfriend, although the prison didn't have any official phone lines for prisoners:

'As I said to you, Mark, I was always needy, always clingy … and I was always on the phone to her. I used to go to the office and beg them to let me call her, because the separation was so intense, I needed to talk to her. They usually let me do that, but I used to tear the arse out of it, making phone call after phone call. After one visit, I came up to the office and asked to use the phone, but the officer just got out the phone log and showed me: call after call after call, in my name, to Jeanne. He said, "No you can't."

'So I picked a pen up off the desk and put it to my throat, and said, "I'm going to do myself": I basically took myself hostage, you know, let me have a phone call or I'll do the loony thing.'

Eddie chuckles about this, perhaps at the idea of anyone threatening themselves with a biro, but although he got his phone call, the staff were not amused: they transferred him to a young offenders' institution with special provision for young men with psychiatric problems. He says there wasn't much in the way of support for mental illness, it wasn't a hospital and he only saw a psychologist once or twice, but it was one of the happier times in his life as the institution was well-stocked with amenities, including a pool table.

However, Jeanne wrote to Eddie when he was about two months from release saying that she was breaking up with him. Eddie says that he didn't make a big deal of this, that the staff took it far more seriously than he did, calling him into a meeting with two senior officers and the matron to solemnly disclose the news that he had been dumped. 'I thought someone had died!' Eddie says to me.

He was duly released back to his mum's house and Jeanne brought the baby around to see him, but Eddie remembers, 'I just didn't feel any connection to her ... like she wasn't really my baby or something. Jeanne said, "Are you going to help me raise this baby?" and I just said, "No."'

Jeanne had another boyfriend, one of the neighbourhood boys, who Eddie really seems to like – 'I just respected him, you know? He was a lovely guy.' – which I think made him something of a rarity as far as the men in Eddie's life went, and they all agreed amicably that it was best if Jeanne and her new partner raised the baby without Eddie's input. If this sounds a bit like a non-story, I think that's the point: Eddie had really seemed to respond well to the time on his own in the YOI, and when he was clean and sober he was capable of being the better man and making life decisions that considered other people's feelings and the greater good, rather than just his own satisfaction. I think this is what makes Eddie likable despite all the bad choices he has made, and the harm he has caused: I get the sense that he has a moral compass, and that he would rather find solutions that work out well for everyone. Unfortunately, as a young man he was rarely sober enough for this moral reasoning to have a chance.

Nothing in Eddie's early life tended to last. Now aged 19 he started another relationship with a woman his own age. Again, he started using drugs and drinking, again his girlfriend became pregnant, and again she ended up giving birth while Eddie was in prison. Eddie had gone out to a party with his male friends and taken a bunch of pills – he didn't know what they were, he'd just taken everything he'd been offered – and sexually assaulted a woman. He had been walking behind her on the way home, caught up and started a conversation with her. They'd approached a park and Eddie had suggested a 'kiss and a cuddle' but she refused. Eddie had put his hand down her top and grabbed her breast. Eddie describes being furious with himself about this, and rightly so: it was a stupid, self-serving crime full of callous entitlement. Not only were convictions for sexual crimes in the 1980s around six times what they are today, but the girl he had attacked was part of the local community. When Eddie was drinking in the pub a few weeks later, her brothers and a group of their friends spotted him, attacked him and then called the police. There had also been a witness: someone had seen Eddie assault the woman and seen her struggle and protest.

Now anyone who has been to prison themselves will attest that there is a very different life for those convicted of sex offences from those with 'normal' (that is to say, violent) offences. There is an implicit hierarchy of crime, with robbers – in my experience, some of the most psychopathic offenders – at the top, followed by violent offenders, then sexual offenders against adults, then grasses or informers, and sexual offenders against children are at the very bottom. Modern jails in Britain usually operate a quasi-segregation system whereby 'vulnerable prisoners' or 'VPs', typically sex offenders plus those who are at risk of harm from other prisoners, are kept in separate wings where the risk against them can be managed. Eddie's previous visits to jail had been as a young offender serving time for theft or violence: an offender at the top of the heap. Now he was a young man in an adult jail for a sexual offence, right down at the bottom. He describes how, on his first reception to the adult prison, the orderlies were serving prisoners: when they asked him to state his index offence and sentence, he refused and they had assumed (correctly) that he was a sex offender and rushed him: five against one.

Scared and deeply ashamed of himself, Eddie took the option of a VP wing for a few weeks, where he began to try to make sense of it all. His solution, not the easiest one but probably the only way to keep himself as the 'good guy' in his life story, was simply to start forcing himself to believe he simply hadn't done it:

'I was saying to myself every night, "I never done it, I never done it." Then when I went to sleep I'd keep hearing it, too: "I never done it." And I ended up believing it, to a certain extent. I decided to go back on the regular wing and told the governor; at the time they couldn't legally keep me on VP so off I went.'

Of course, infected with this combination of toxic masculinity, self-delusion and a regular supply of cannabis sourced from his brothers, who had set themselves up as dealers, Eddie's first order of business was to get revenge on the inmates who had attacked him at reception. He bided his time until he caught one of them alone in his cell with the door open, then charged in. Here's Eddie's account:

'We started having a punch-up, and I just bit onto his ear. The bell went off – someone must have heard the commotion – and the screws came in, lifted me up, and I'm there with my teeth still on his earhole. They said, "You're gonna have to let go or we'll hit you with the truncheons," so I let go and they carried me down the block. I got a week down the block, lost earnings, but then I got back on the wing and all the fellas [that attacked me] were coming up to me saying, "Oh, it was nothing to do with me." I'm not trying to give the impression I was really dangerous. I was scared, scared of talking to people, scared of interacting ... but I *was* up for it, and they knew I was up for it; so they just got themselves shipped out.'

I didn't get the impression here that Eddie was trying to big himself up: I think he was a bit incredulous at the way his plan, namely 'convince yourself you didn't assault that woman, and go after the guys that think you did so they can't tell anyone else', had worked out. It was almost like a perfect reinforcement of every violent, aggressive, guilt-denying, victim-blaming impulse Eddie

had had inside himself. Having established himself as a top dog, Eddie went on to make good in
the adult prison: he developed a good relationship
with the officers, started a job on the hotplate (a
coveted role, as food is perhaps the most important commodity in prison after contraband) and
the attacks stopped. For a while. Of course, this
being Eddie, it was only temporary: after a few
months of relative peace, he tipped a tea urn over
another prisoner who had taken umbrage at the
way Eddie poured his cuppa, and off went Eddie
to another prison.

I have met a lot of men like the young Eddie:
men for whom prison is not a quiet place to 'do
your bird and keep your head down' in the words
of one lifer (who, ironically, was terrible at keeping
his own advice and was constantly in segregation),
but rather something between a Roman gladiator-
ial ring and an opportunity to get your own back
against 'the system'. I do understand why Eddie
himself was so angry with men in positions of
power – from his biological father to his mother's
third husband to the prison officers who allowed

him to be shamed and assaulted in reception, they had let him down again and again. However, this grievance attitude to prison has a real danger that the prisoner becomes like Charles Salvador, a.k.a. Charles Bronson, the British robber who was originally sentenced to seven years in 1974 but has spent his entire life behind bars. Bronson is now serving a life sentence because of his repeated attacks on prison officers and prison property.

Prison is a hard place, no doubt: but it can get inside some angry young men's heads and become a far worse place than it is intended to be: an internal prison that they are forever trying to break out of while losing sight of what it means to be free. I was horrified to find out recently that a young man I worked with in the early 2000s, who had been given a five-year sentence for GBH, was still in institutions: he had been transferred to a secure hospital and there caused so much damage and disturbance that the psychiatrists felt he was unsafe to release. Now in his fifties, he had recently had a stroke – although the hospital was moving to release him, he was quite frail and there are concerns that he might not be able to manage living in society again.

Fortunately, despite his transgressive behaviour, Eddie managed to escape any further sanctions or prison time. When he was released after 16 months inside, Eddie's life followed a pretty similar pattern to the previous time. Again, he met his new child, a boy, and made up with his girlfriend, but once again they agreed to go their separate ways and Eddie moved on to a new woman. Part of me wonders if maybe taking on the responsibilities of a father might have settled Eddie down a bit and got him away from drink, drugs and crime, but then I think about how worryingly close the younger Eddie's controlling, aggressive behaviour sometimes came to that of his stepfather. That part of me starts to worry for any child to be around such unpredict-ability, and perhaps this was just the way things had to be, as Eddie crashed from bad situation to worse situation.

To make money, Eddie had settled into a very lucrative job acting as a 'hoister' – a professional shoplifter – of designer clothes from big department stores. He was, for once, making good money and was well-dressed. Then, Eddie and his girlfriend went out drinking and smoking, and on the way back from the pub they had a disagreement with a group of girls also walking down the street. Words were exchanged, and one of the girls ran off and returned with her father, a man Eddie knew from his days of boosting goods at the docks, together with his stepson, Jimmy, who was packing a knife and started threatening Eddie.

Someone – he doesn't remember who – passed Eddie a knife of his own, and he set off after the men down the street back to their house. The men closed the door in his face, to which Eddie responded by throwing a garden gnome through the window. The father and Jimmy came running out at Eddie, armed with a knife and baseball bat respectively, and chased him back down the street. Then the unthinkable happened: Jimmy took a swing at Eddie, who ducked the blow and tripped, sending the hand holding his own knife flying out backwards. Jimmy overbalanced, having missed, and fell chest-first onto the knife, which penetrated his heart. Suddenly, Eddie was responsible for the death of one of his childhood friends.

I don't know whether anyone would have been hurt that evening if Eddie had not tripped. The way he told it, it sounded like most of the evening was just regular bravado and posturing, and once again it was that extra bit of bad luck in a risky situation that turned Eddie into a killer. Although the prosecution initially argued for murder, there was no evidence to support that charge and the jury found Eddie guilty of manslaughter. He was given a five-year sentence.

I know from reading many newspaper articles about killers that the general public dislike feeling empathy for the perpetrator. In Eddie's case, though, it sounds as though the knowledge of what he had done – taken a life after a pointless argument – affected him terribly. He battled with it internally, trying to keep up the facade of a tough guy, of a psychopath who didn't care about what he'd done:

'There were times within my prison sentence when I felt quite happy to be in that category, "I've taken someone's life", like a chest-out thing. But when I let it come to me and thought about it and thought about it, it devastated me.'

This sentence was not a good one for Eddie. He had started to develop psychotic symptoms consistent with post-traumatic stress disorder, probably worsened by the high-grade cannabis his brothers were still sending him. The combination of drugs and trauma led him to start experiencing delusional parasitosis: a condition where someone believes they are infested with insects or bugs, spiders in Eddie's case, which caused him to scratch his head and pull out his hair. Also, because of the drugs, he became known as a troublemaker within the prison and he was frequently in conflict with the officers. Eddie explains one incident:

'I was on one wing that was full of psychos, the nut-nut [psychiatric] wing. It's supposed to be a medical wing, but if you fuck up on the normal wing, they'd put you there, because it was horrific. One morning I was having a shave, and it was back in the day when you had to share the razors – they stored them in some solution, but it was still dangerous [for catching bloodborne infections].

'Anyway, I did half my face, and then I started getting all cut. So I went to the screw: "Here, can I have a new blade, it's cutting me to bits, look," and he just says, "No you can't, you have to use that one." I said, "Come on, be fair; I've got a visit this afternoon," but he just said, "No." So I said, "Alright, I'll just finish up with this one then," and he said, "No you won't; shaving's finished now." So I walk out and I've only got half a beard. So they're pushing me down the landing, jostling me, and I just turn around and flobbed [spat] in one of their faces.

'That was it: I was dragged down the metal stairs, put in a solitary cell and had a pot of piss thrown over me, because it was back in the days when we still slopped out [until the 1990s, prisoners had to use buckets for urine and faeces] and I was in there for three or four days.'

At the end of this he was offered the chance to go to HMP Grendon, a therapeutic community that is a place where prisoners who want to change their lives can receive psychological treatment for their offending, but unfortunately Eddie only had a few months left to serve on his sentence and the community decided this wasn't long enough for him to do the work he needed. Perhaps they were right, but this meant that Eddie received only short-term, medical treatment for his symptoms: clunky and only partly effective anti-psychotic medication. Then he was released without any further support.

'When you take a life, it has a huge effect on you. It hurt me. Obviously, it hurt the boy's family more, but still, it damaged me. When I came out I was 25 and an angry young man. I started drinking again, puffing and thieving ... I came back to Docklands, but I felt in danger over all the things I'd done.'

Scared of the consequences of his crimes against members of the Docklands community, Eddie moved around the country, eventually settling in Southend. Fundamentally, he was without help and unable to get out of repeating the same cycles: drinking, smoking, stealing and getting into relationships with women whose own instability and promiscuity was like a red rag to a bull for Eddie. The relationships would turn violent, with Eddie nearly always having the last word and sometimes badly hurting his partners in the process.

One of his only stable points in this was perhaps Janine, a woman from Docklands who had taken a shine to Eddie since they were teenagers and with whom he'd had an on/off relationship for many years. Unlike a lot of the other women he had been involved with, Janine seemed to be a calming and stable influence on Eddie: he had met her parents, who liked him, and he'd never engaged with her in the fights and abuse that had plagued his other relationships.

When Eddie was about 30, things were going particularly badly for him in Southend, and he came back to his mum's in Docklands to try to regroup. A letter from Janine was there waiting for him and he gave her a call. They spent some time together, and after a few days she suggested he come over to her parents' house for dinner, saying, 'I've got something to show you.' Curious, Eddie came over to her place and she took him upstairs and told him, 'I've become a prison officer; look, here's the uniform.'

Eddie was taken aback. Not only had the two of them shared more than just the occasional spliff, but Eddie was a convicted criminal. His relationship with prison officers in general was difficult, to say the least: for every reasonable officer he had worked with, there was another 'screw' who he felt had messed with him or abused their power over him in some way.

I don't fully understand Janine's motives for telling Eddie this about herself; perhaps she thought that he would inevitably be back in prison and was preparing for the worst, but even then I don't think she could have ever imagined how bad things would get. To start with, things between Janine and Eddie cooled a bit and she stopped returning his calls. Shortly afterwards, Janine moved into a flat with another female officer, Sonia, to save money.

Christmas Eve came around and Eddie, feeling lonely, went around to Janine's place to find her. Sonia answered the door and said that Janine was out, so Eddie suggested that they go for a Christmas drink together. Sonia agreed, so they had three or four drinks in the pub, chatting happily, and then he walked Sonia back to the flat. When they got back, Eddie asked, 'Listen, can I come up and use the phone to call Janine at her parents'?' Sonia said she wasn't sure, but in the days before mobile phones she perhaps thought it would be unfair to make Eddie walk home just to make a call, so she agreed, perhaps reluctantly, and they went upstairs together to the bedroom where the phone was.

When they got upstairs, though, Eddie told me he went from wanting to make the call to a very different set of thoughts. He remembers feeling angry at Janine for freezing him out, scared of women he couldn't ever seem to make a proper relationship with and angry with prison officers for the way he'd been treated in his last sentence. He grabbed at Sonia and told her he wanted to have sex. Sonia said no, and Eddie said that he remembered being overwhelmed by pure hatred.

'You cunts fucked me right about, and I always said I'd get my revenge, so this is it.'

Eddie forced a petrified Sonia down on the bed and raped her.

Eddie ran off to Southend and drank himself into a haze. When he was arrested a few days later for robbing a man in the street – for £4, he recalls – the police identified him as wanted for the rape. He intended to plead not guilty, but Sonia's statement was persuasive – bold, detailed and plausible – so Eddie went for guilty and was given a nine-year sentence. Suddenly he was in the care of prison officers again, one of whose best friend he had raped.

To the credit of prison officers everywhere, however, aside from being moved around a lot, Eddie was never victimised. 'They were professional, and they stuck to it,' he said. Eddie still had a very wayward approach to prison life: he continued to deal cannabis and extort other prisoners who wouldn't pay, and was placed in segregation for 13 months in a single stretch, a length of time that was made illegal shortly after, in 2004. He doesn't hold a grudge though: this was the game he had chosen to play during his sentence.

There's a long pause on the tape after Eddie tells me the story of the rape, as I try to make sense of it. My first thought was, why did he not just wait for Janine to come back if he wanted sex? But I was wrong here. Most rape isn't about sex, it's about something else: about revenge and control. Eddie told me that when he said 'you cunts' to Sonia he meant prison officers, but I think that it could equally have meant women; or anyone in authority throughout his life. None of this excuses what he did, and Eddie is the first person to admit this, but understanding and forgiving are different things. I also felt angry and frustrated at the younger Eddie, making the same mistakes over, and over and over, and never learning. At the same time, though, I thought: did nobody ever think to offer him some help? One of the great difficulties of personality disorders is that they tend to be 'ego syntonic', a fancy way of saying that people with a diagnosis of these disorders don't often think that there's anything wrong at all.

Eddie had come within a hair's breadth of being admitted to a treatment programme at Grendon for his offending but had missed out because of a technicality. Instead he had gone on to repeat his destructive cycle of minor crime, drug and alcohol abuse, meeting a partner who was poorly matched for him, starting a relationship that was too intense to last, then finally committing a serious crime that sent him to prison, where he continued taking and dealing drugs. I believe that there is evidence from Eddie's past that this is a surprisingly fragile cycle of events: take away one aspect, be it alcohol, drugs in prison or the relationship, and the whole chain is preventable. Nobody in a position of authority seemed to realise this, however, and combined with Eddie's natural distrust of anyone in authority – the controlling 'sergeant majors' – he was never offered the help he needed.

*

As it happened, help for Eddie did finally come. He was 37 when he left prison after being found guilty of rape; it was 20 years after his first prison sentence. He told me he remembered walking around south London one day feeling 'murderous', like he was 'in a lot of trouble' and might seriously hurt someone. He noticed that as he walked around train stations, people recoiled to get out of his way, as though he looked like he might lash out at any moment. He felt like he had become so many things that he hated – he had nothing, had lost so many relationships and now he had the knowledge that he had it in him to rape another person – and he booked himself an appointment at the local mental health clinic and asked for help. He was referred to the forensic psychotherapy service in Hackney to work with Dr C., a noted consultant psychotherapist who worked in a psychoanalytic way.

Hearing Eddie describe this now, I am struck by how easy it was for him to get help the moment he asked for it. I'm also reminded of the many young men I have worked with who have asked for this same kind of help in the last ten to fifteen years but been rebuffed by mental health trusts because there are so few forensic outpatient services remaining.

Very quickly after starting weekly sessions with Dr C., things started to change for Eddie. He stopped getting routinely involved with crime, started to avoid violent situations and finally started to think through his interactions with other people. He met another woman, Tina, and managed to sustain his longest ever relationship. Finally, it looked as though the cycle had been broken for Eddie, but then fate intervened again. His mother became very unwell, and after a year-long illness, during which Eddie had moved back to be with her, she died in her home in Docklands.

One of the most interesting phenomena of classical behavioural psychology is something called the 'extinction burst';[2] this is something that happens as an organism (a human or any other animal) is on the verge of giving up on a learned behaviour. For a brief period, the frequency of the behaviour that is going 'extinct'[3] shows a 'burst' of frequency, almost as if it is raging against its inevitable loss, as the organism tries one last time to get the reward it used to with the behaviour. In Eddie's case, this meant that after his mother's death his antisocial tendencies suddenly made a ferocious comeback. He started 'hoisting' again and doing drugs with his partner. Worse yet, he tried to hide this behaviour from Dr C. because he felt ashamed, promising instead that everything was fine.

His relationship with Tina became unstable, full of dramatic (if not violent) arguments, and they started to get into the on/off cycle that had characterised his relationship with Janine. One night, Eddie went out and got steaming drunk, and when he returned to the flat they shared, Tina – perhaps not unreasonably – refused to let him in. He started shouting, and she shouted back, and since this was getting nowhere, he asked Tina to at least throw him the car keys so he could go somewhere else for the night. She did, but not before calling the police: although we'll never know if this was out of a protective instinct for herself or for Eddie, who was about to drive his car while blind drunk.

Sure enough, the moment Eddie got in his car, the police showed up and started to pursue him. In almost a reflex, Eddie went faster and faster to escape, but then lost control while doing 120mph and hit a sloped crash barrier in the middle of the road that flipped his car up and over a round-about into a wall on the opposite side. The impact smashed Eddie's pelvis in five places and put him in intensive care for three months. Tina dumped him while he was still confined to his bed, although they did agree to remain friends.

Recovery from the accident was slow and dif-ficult, and one of the side effects was that Eddie had several complex hernias from where intes-tinal tissue had pushed through the weakened area around his pelvis. He had to have another oper-ation to treat this, and while he was recovering, he met Sara – a recent divorcee – who was an out-patient. They got on very well, and Sara invited him to visit her on her farm in Dorset. Eddie – show-ing remarkably persistent dedication to the cause of doomed intimate relationships – hitchhiked all the way from Docklands to Dorset with a barely healed pelvis.

We know the plot of this movie, though. Sara was wealthy, independent and enjoying her life, and had no intentions of being monogamous with a man who lived more than 100 miles away. She was seeing other men and wasn't making much of an effort to hide it, so Eddie found out and, inevitably, 'hit the roof'. At least he managed to refrain from physically hurting Sara, but instead humiliated her by pouring a bucket of ice-cold water over her. Sara didn't take kindly to this and told the police, who pressed a common assault charge against Eddie. Common assault, unlike assault occasioning actual bodily harm, is not usually punished with prison time in the UK, but Eddie was classed as a 'dangerous offender' as a result of his previous convictions, meaning it was treated as seriously as possible and he was given a two-year prison sentence.

When he told me this story, I noticed that Eddie's face was contorted into an expression of complete contempt; he was furious with himself. I told him this, and he said:

'I was devastated, you know. At the time I felt I was living the dream: my own house, drinking and smoking when I wanted. The money I had, the freedom I had ... and I'd just thrown it all away. All of a sudden I was going to lose my house, my freedom, my self-respect ... I was just disgusted with myself. I just thought, "My fucking life's finished." So I did the only thing I could, I wrote to Dr C. from prison.'

As it happens, I know Dr C. very well; she was the lead therapist on a couple of the cases I have described already. She does not suffer fools gladly and usually takes colossal fuck-ups of the scale that Eddie had just committed very seriously. So she must have really seen something in Eddie worth persevering with, because she came to see him in prison and recommend a transfer to a secure hospital where she worked under the Mental Health Act. This hospital offered a therapeutic community model, like Grendon prison, where Eddie would be forced to work on his offending behaviour, as well as his anger and violent, controlling behaviour. Unlike Dr C.'s outpatient clinic, he wouldn't be able to leave the secure hospital to hoist goods, meet women or to make up stories about what he was up to the night before. He would still have to serve out his sentence, but while he did that he would have to face up to his problems or be sent back to prison. Eddie made a good decision: he agreed to Dr C.'s offer to move to the hospital. He confessed to me:

'I was sort of in two minds, I wanted to change, I was disgusted with myself, but at the same time I sort of wanted an easy ride. It was only when I got there that I realised it wasn't, it wasn't at all. It's changed my life, and I'm constantly surprised I'm not doing a life sentence, and it's mostly because of Dr C. and the unit.'

I asked Eddie what he thought made the therapeutic community approach work for him.

'I would walk around the unit and hear all these people shouting and moaning, kicking off, and I thought: that's exactly how I was. But I also saw people change from that place, and I wanted to do that too. I think I came to see that I was in pain, all the time, and Dr C. and the others showed me empathy, compassion, but also were straight up with me: why did I always have to have all these drugs inside me to speak to other people? And why did it always have to be me sitting inside the prison cell? I would want to go on the rampage and she'd just ask me: "Well, why does it have to be you who's the one who does that?" And that just made me think, you know, "Why should it be me? Why not someone else for once?"'

All this took place nearly 20 years ago now. Eddie finished his sentence, was discharged from the secure unit and even his sessions with Dr C. have come to an end. He has been in the same relationship for the last nine years, and says his life is both happy and normal. As he and I finished our second round of cakes after our final interview session, I was inclined to agree, and at the same time I thought we were both a bit relieved and amazed to have made it through his history. I asked Eddie what the word 'psychopath' meant to him:

'Dr C. explained to me that a psychopath is someone does things off the social norm. But I would say a psychopath is someone who's a raving lunatic, who goes around stabbing people or hurting people, and I have done that, but someone who has no feelings about it. Some of the thoughts and feelings I did get, I still get, but I push them away: I just think it's not worth it. I used to let the thoughts build but now I have to close them off. I don't know if you can develop empathy, but I believe I have. I mean, there have been times when I just didn't give a fuck; I had no empathy for anyone.'

Is Eddie really a psychopath? Officially he is: he has the Psychopathy Test results to prove it and has spent time in a service specially designed for men with that diagnosis, which in the end transformed his life for the better. He has spent 16 years of his life in prison, including time for manslaughter, actual bodily harm and rape: very serious crimes that it is hard to believe anyone with a shred of empathy would ever have committed.

As I explained to Eddie, though, I think that he developed a psychopathic persona, a defence, in response to the brutality of his childhood with his mother's third husband. I think that, for Eddie, coming to believe that everyone else was undeserving of love or respect, and everything had to be about getting what he wanted, was the only way to protect himself and make sense of his family's victimisation at the hands of a man who sounds manipulative, aggressive and controlling: the traits of a psychopath. Had his mother stayed with Martin, for example, I am sure that Eddie would still have got into trouble a lot when he was younger, but I think that over time this would have faded away and he could have led a fulfilling life outside of prison.

So for me, Eddie's psychopathy is only surface-deep. He has shown a lack of remorse and empathy, he has broken the law, been aggressive, a juvenile delinquent, a serial monogamist, occasionally leeching off his partners, and someone who has been unable to control his behaviour. What he isn't, though, is any kind of Machiavellian like Paul or

Tony. He is not a pathological liar, although he has certainly told some whoppers, and he's not grandiose or superficially charming. In fact, he comes across as a bit prickly at first, and it takes a while to warm up to him; almost the exact opposite of Tony's oozy charm. Sometimes I struggled to match Eddie's current empathy with his terrible past, but unlike a lot of offenders I have worked with he doesn't just tell me he has changed: he shows me. He talks about his particular shame for raping Sonia when, 'she was lovely to me, she never did me any harm'. When we got to the equally difficult subject of his relationship with his mother after the abuse from her third husband, Eddie told me: 'I've sat here with my mum and talked about it. She thought I hated her for it, and I told her no, no … now I'm older I understand that she was living in fear.'

What also strikes me about Eddie is that he jumped at the first real offer of help he received, and it changed his life. Yes, he nearly fucked it up along the way, but every psychologist knows about the Stages of Change theory[4] – that even after we start to change our fundamental behaviours there will be lapses on the way to maintaining them permanently, and that is normal. It's just that Eddie's behaviour was so extreme, and he was so locked into this destructive downward spiral of relationships with his partners, that perhaps we should be relieved that – while unacceptable – his last aggressive act was to inflict humiliation and discomfort with the water bucket rather than physical injury.

I'm not sure that Eddie's pathway to happiness, a crime-free life and the ability to have civilised conversation with a former prison psychologist over coffee and cakes would work for every case in this book, let alone all psychopaths, although I wish that was the case. But it does remind me that there is always hope, and that sometimes it is just the offer of real help, help that means talking about the difficult stuff and not just dishing out platitudes and medication, that is the most important thing. It is so easy to write off an angry, violent young man as a lost cause, as an untreatable psychopath, as so many people did throughout Eddie's life, and forget that nobody is defined entirely by being a psychopath: there is always an individual human being with a history, wants and needs underneath that callous exterior. If we forget that, we forget how and why to have hope.

Chapter Nine
Psychopathy is Bad for your Health

Looking back, I'm struck by how dark some of these stories are; far darker than they exist in my working memory where I tend to 'edit out' some of the nastier bits, probably to make the recollections easier to live with. The hardest part of some of the stories is the sense of tragedy: if only this small thing had been different, none of this might have happened. I chose to finish the case studies with Eddie, not because it was one of the few positive stories – fortunately there have been many positive endings in my experience – but because Eddie's criminal history was relatively serious, and in general it is those men with the most serious histories who find it hardest to make changes. What is also unique about Eddie is that despite his complex and extensive offending history, and a history of severe mental illness as well as psychopathy, he could change the direction of his life while he still had time to live it. I learned a lot from interviewing him for this book, but while he gave me a lot of hope, he puts cases like Danny and Tony, where I couldn't see a happy ending, into sharp contrast.

I said in the introduction that I wanted to write a book about how diverse and complex psychopaths are, how ineffective we are at understanding and rehabilitating them, and perhaps also start the process of trying to rehumanise people's perceptions of psychopaths and their stories. Whatever the endless spew of articles in popular magazines might say, psychopaths are not something you should routinely worry about. I get it: nobody wants to inadvertently start a relationship with a psychopath. But, as we have seen, psychopaths are not people whom it is easy to be in a relationship with. It very quickly becomes clear when a potential partner is not interested in your emotional fulfilment, or much else about you at all. This is a good sign – not restricted to dating psychopaths – that you should probably leave that relationship and take your chances elsewhere, and if you do not then there are probably things in your own mind that should be a higher priority for you to address than your partner's mental health issues.

Psychopaths don't have a monopoly on manipulation and bullying, nor do people with narcissistic or borderline personality disorder. Nor is it easy even for someone very experienced and skilled at making these kind of distinctions always to tell whether someone is a 'vulnerable narcissist' or an 'aggressive borderline' – so you should be very wary when reading an article that tells you that these are the kind of people you should avoid on the dating scene. If you start to learn how to tell them apart, call my boss and you can have my job.

There are many creative attempts by academics and some clinicians to move the discussion about psychopathy away from criminality and the Psychopathy Test and into community psychology and psychiatry. This is helpful, because there are a fair number of people in the community who would not meet the criteria for criminal psychopathy on the PCL-R, but do have a lot of the emotional (or 'affective') and interpersonal features that make up a major part of psychopathy: lack of remorse, pathological lying, glib and superficial charm, conning and manipulative; but none of the antisocial elements. These are often called 'successful psychopaths' – successful in the dual sense of both 'succeeding at life' but also perhaps in 'not having been caught doing anything criminal' – and may make up 3.5 per cent of people in the business world[1]. How concerned should you be about a 'psychopath' who is no more likely than a non-psychopath to commit violence? Certainly, 'successful' psychopaths are often experts in relational aggression – bullying, controlling behaviour designed to damage people's social status[2] – but there is also some evidence that these people are different from criminal psychopaths in fundamental aspects of their brain function. As well as a higher IQ, in some studies higher than the population average,[3] and less impairment in the areas of their brain typically associated with criminal psychopathy, they often have high levels of 'cognitive empathy', that is, the ability to recognise emotion in others without feeling it.[4]

I have two problems with this argument. First, my clinical experience says that some 'successful' psychopaths do indeed make it into the criminal justice system: this is why I picked Tony as a case study. Anyone who can set up a fraudulent business empire, including a credit union, and also survive in high-security conditions surrounded by murderers and so-called 'unsuccessful' psychopaths, must have an abnormally high level of cunning, at least. So 'successful' psychopaths are not necessarily defined by evading capture, and don't take my word for it: watch one of disgraced banker Nick Leeson's post-prison interviews where he – very effectively – assigns blame for all his criminal negligence to the way he was managed and the culture in the bank where he worked. Defining the adaptability of someone's disorder in relation to the highly complex social question of whether they are detected and punished for it seems a bit arbitrary, to say the least.

But my second problem with the idea that psychopaths are broadly 'successful' or 'unsuccessful' is more logical than experiential: I don't know if two people who are different in terms of their neurophysiology, executive function and emotional reasoning are really the same type of person, or whether they can both meaningfully be given the same label, whether that's 'psychopath' or something else altogether. Sure, I wouldn't particularly want to work for a so-called 'successful' psychopath, but I'd take that over working for someone like Paul on any day of the week, month, year or century. In fact, I think I'd really like to work with James Fallon at Stanford (Hi, Jim!), but we'll come back to him later.

Part of the reason we're so preoccupied with psychopaths is that the media are always leading the way on it for us. Frustratingly, discussions of psychopathy in the press are almost always inaccurate; it's pointless giving out the list of 20 items on the psychopathy test *yet again* to fill up space on a newspaper page when anyone who uses the test needs to have either a PhD or extensive clinical training, go on a three-day course explicitly accredited by Robert Hare himself, and complete a set of case studies to within an acceptable level of accuracy. Having the list of psychopathic traits on their own without the highly copyrighted rubric describing them is like having a list of the component parts of the *Discovery* shuttle – well, at least a Volkswagen Beetle – you can try to put them together without expert help but what comes out is most likely going to be a confusing mess.

Even when the press feature interviews with experts, the articles can end up being misleading. Different theoretical perspectives – psychoanalytic, neurocognitive, genetic – are presented as the same thing, but they have a surprisingly large number of disagreements about where psychopathy comes from and the best way to address it. One of the biggest issues, which isn't by any means unique to psychopathy – I've moaned about it applying to narcissism just as much[5] – is that lots of researchers will give out semi-validated (meaning that they showed some base-level agreement with the Psychopathy Test in one study) self-report questionnaires to a sample of college students and use this to deduce fundamental truths about psychopaths. Universities issue a press release with the word 'psychopath' and the media get excited.

But we wouldn't confuse 'people who feel tired' (or parents, as we are usually known) with 'chronic fatigue syndrome' because, if we did, the diagnosis wouldn't have any meaning. Why are we so keen to accept this with psychopathy? It makes sense that psychopathy should be a continuum, sure, but there is some convincing evidence that actually asking psychopaths – who, let us not forget, are supposed to be pathological liars – about their psychopathy is very different to measuring it using a checklist based on professional judgement.[6] Perhaps the take-home message is that our understanding of psychopathy has developed tremendously

Some of the most useful, well-conducted research on psychopaths comes from geneticists and genetic epidemiologists such as Essi Viding, who found that children with high levels of callous and unemotional traits that can predict adult psychopathy often have a similar genetic profile.[7] But I don't think that criminal psychopaths ever come from stable, safe 'good enough' homes and families. Genetic heritage, or 'character', is an important factor, but it is the environment the child grows up in that makes the difference. James Fallon has the genes and the brain of a psychopath, sure, but he isn't a risk to anyone and his contribution to society is far more valuable than the fact he's a bit distant with his kids and wishes annoying dinner guests would 'fuck off'. So although I think that an overhaul of the terminology, diagnostic process and treatment of psychopathy is long, long overdue, I also think that in some ways it's helpful that psychopathy is mostly shackled to criminal behaviour by the PCL-R. I can accept this is scientifically problematic, but morally it is far more palatable than landing a quasi-clinical and highly stigmatising diagnosis on people like Jim.

None of this means that criminal psychopaths are not culpable for what they do. Part of the journey into change is the acceptance and understanding that what you did was wrong and ultimately you are accountable for it, just as it was for Eddie. However, I believe forensic psychology and psychiatry are often insufficiently attentive to social context, particularly in the English-speaking countries that offer rehabilitative services to psychopaths. We tend to think of psychopathy, and other mental disorders, in very biomedical terms that suggest that if we just have the right magic pill (or psychotherapy or managed clinical team) we can solve the problem. Other countries are a lot less grandiose about this, and a lot more pragmatic. In the Netherlands, for example, offenders with a diagnosis of personality disorder are assigned to a single clinic, usually close to their home, that provides care and rehabilitation for them throughout their entire sentence.

I have visited a few of these clinics but I particularly remember going to the Van der Hoeven Kliniek in Utrecht in 2005. Although it was originally set up by a psychiatrist, since the 1990s the Van der Hoeven has been run not by a psychiatrist, psychologist or sociologist, but by an economist. Although it provides a public service of rehabilitating mentally disordered offenders underwritten by the Dutch Ministry of Justice, everything it does seeks to be completely cost-neutral to the public. This means that, when I visited, the café, restaurant and reception desk were all run by patients with criminal histories. The centre of the clinic housed a massive workshop where patients worked on real, private manufacturing contracts producing, among other things, electric forklifts, circuit boards and stitched leather goods, for which they were paid a real wage. When patients reduced their risk enough to move on from being inpatients confined to the hospital, they were given a flat in a building near to the clinic so that they could continue to attend the workshop and any therapy sessions they still needed.

To demonstrate the strength of this model, the staff of the clinic played a very Dutch trick on me. Or at least, I think it was a trick; perhaps they just didn't realise there was anything weird about it at all. While I was visiting one of the wards, or living blocks, I attended what I thought was a meeting of patients – all with a diagnosis of personality disorder or psychopathy plus a serious offending history – together with a couple of staff members. Throughout the meeting a couple of patients got up and left, but this happens in my clinical sessions all the time, so I didn't think too much of it. It was only when the meeting finished and everyone got up to leave that I realised that there were absolutely no staff members in the group at all: they had been the ones who had left earlier, probably because they realised everything was fine and they weren't really needed. One of the women I had thought was a staff member had in fact burned both her parents to death in their own bed when she was a teenager.

As if to ram the message home, there was even a small incident on the (mixed) ward later that day where a couple of male patients had a disagreement, and one of them started to become aggressive. In a British hospital the alarm would have sounded, and a team of specially trained nurses would have sailed in to restrain the patient and take him to a seclusion ward away from the others. In the Van der Hoeven, it was a team of patients who calmly asked the man to accompany them to the de-escalation room. Which he did. At the evening handover one of the staff nonchalantly described the aggressive patient as a 'violent psychopath', as if it was no big thing.

On my last day in Utrecht I had a brief meeting with the lead psychiatrist and psychologist while walking around the park that made up the central area of the main clinic. I told them that their clinic was amazing – which from their reaction they already seemed to be well aware of – and I asked them where the inspiration for the model came from. I wished I hadn't asked: the psychiatrist chuckled and said to me, 'Well, we visited the Henderson Hospital in the 1950s and we borrowed a lot of the ideas from that.' The Henderson, of course, was a psychiatric unit that catered for men and women with personality disorders that was opened in 1947[8] and then closed in 2008 when the NHS reorganisation meant that primary care trusts could no longer fund out-of-area care for their patients. The British invented this model – what we would call a therapeutic community, the same placement that helped Eddie so much, where the hierarchy between staff and patients is radically diminished – and now seem to have all but forgotten it.

Why is this story about the Dutch clinic so important? I think this about 'normal' or 'good enough' human development and how few, if any, psychopaths have experienced anything like it in their lifetimes. Although they may not have any frame of reference for fundamental ideas such as love, compassion and empathy, we cannot infantilise and re-parent psychopathic patients. Instead we must offer a place where they have the opportunity to discover the worth and meaning of these concepts for themselves.

There is strong emerging evidence that if you can intervene early enough, even children with the most appalling histories of neglect, abuse and trauma can experience normal neurodevelopment and 'prevent' psychopathy.[9] For some men and women, such as Eddie, the experience of even a limited kind of care can be transformative; for others, the Pauls and Jasons of this world, perhaps the best we can hope for is that they are able to offer a more developed kind of cognitive empathy so they can at least identify emotions in others, if not share them.

Although the evidence is still confused and there is a lot of pessimism, and I think that a lot of this is because we are dead set on finding a single 'magic pill' for psychopathy, whether that be a literal pill as we have for schizophrenia, or a psychological therapy, as we now have with cognitive behavioural therapy (CBT) for depression. Because psychopathy has a complex causality, involving genes, environment, and neuropsychology, it's likely that only a complex treatment will be effective. So, this means focusing on creating an environment that allows for healthy development to take place and avoids re-traumatisation of the kind men like Danny and women in most secure settings seem to experience daily.

Psychopaths need help. Throwing away the key or, worse yet, executing psychopaths as some states in the USA do because their brain doesn't work like it 'should', is pretty monstrous if we consider ourselves a society where psychopaths are supposed to be different precisely because they lack empathy with other humans. Churchill once said that a society's attitude to its prisoners was a measure of its 'stored-up strength', its resolve to provide leeway for people to fail and return, like Eddie, and not be simply cast aside because of their transgressions.

As world-leading psychopath expert James Blair put it in 2013, they 'deserve to be helped',[10] and we are failing both offenders with psychopathic disorder and their victims if we continue to lack an effective framework for helping them. It *is* possible to support them to make better decisions and become better, functioning members of society.

A corollary of this is that work with psychopaths is not nearly recognised enough. Some of the experiences I have told you about, particularly my work with the young man known in this book as Danny, affected me quite profoundly, and not always in a good way. This work has, at times, given me nightmares, physical symptoms and terrible anxiety disorder. And yet hundreds of forensic psychiatrists

and psychologists, nurses, prison officers, proba-
tion officers and social workers go to work with
psychopaths every day of the year.

Most of the time they are expected just to get
on with it, without proper training or a working
clinical model, let alone fuss or recognition. They
need proper supervision and support and a better
understanding of the long-term effects of the work.
Firing and criminalising workers who were manipulated by psychopaths does nobody any favours:
this is a failure of the systems that are supposed
to support workers to do their jobs effectively and
keep them safe.

Psychoanalysts call the staff team working
around severely disordered men and women a
'container':[11] a space that 'contains' the disordered
behaviour and in doing so allows for change and
understanding by their patients, and in the case of
those who have committed crimes, a space that pro-
tects society too. Yet this container is not effective
or safe without proper design and maintenance. In
short, without the recognition that staff working
in prisons and mental hospitals need a great deal

of specific relational support and training, everyone is at risk.

I left clinical work with offenders with a diagnosis of psychopathy in 2015. Since then, my research has moved into questions about how we can understand and prevent violence by understanding its causes. In this bigger picture, psychopathy is not that big a deal. My colleagues and I constructed a machine-learning algorithm that modelled the causes of violence. After major risk factors such as untreated severe mental illness, male gender, anger, previous violence and violent ideation, psychopathy did not even make the top ten most important factors related to whether someone was going to be violent.

Psychopathy is a one-size-fits-all template that provides just one contributory factor for why some people do terrible things and by its nature doesn't get close to explaining the who, when and why of violent crime. Psychopathy isn't like a disorder like erotomania where the victim and the motivation are always the same. (The erotomaniac falls in love with their victim and forms a delusional belief that the victim loves them back, despite any evidence to the contrary. Anyone who threatens this belief – the victim's real partners, usually – is at risk of anything from abuse to murder.) Psychopathy doesn't deal with motivations: in many respects it is unsatisfying as an explanation for anything, but that's because it wasn't designed that way: Cleckley thought it was a way of diagnosing why some of his clients were particularly difficult to work with, and Bob Hare thought it was a way of understanding why some prisoners are so difficult to rehabilitate. Layers of academic research, mythology and media conjecture have buried these relatively humble origins.

All the psychopaths I have worked with have, I believe, been 'made' by an early experience of life that was deeply and profoundly wrong in some important way: parents who were not 'good enough' for their children because they were too focused on their own lives; abusers who were allowed into the family network; and/or a care system that simply couldn't contain the disordered behaviour of these young men and, in some cases, women. Yet it is increasingly being found that the right kind of support offered to young people with antisocial and disordered behaviour can be transformative: multisystemic therapy, that works on the boundaries between families, schools and the police to keep children and young adults out of prison;[12] intensive interventions targeted at specific patterns of abuse.[13] The problem is not that we have no way of helping people, it is that when someone does not know that they should seek help, as Eddie didn't until it was almost too late, we are very bad at seeing past the denials and minimisations of pain to make that first bold offer. It's bold because we might well know, or at least suspect, that it will be thrown back in our faces when we do.

Psychopathy as a concept and a diagnosis is at once complex and reductive: it describes a lack, an absence of something – a belief that other people have value in their own right – that a healthy individual draws great richness and satisfaction from every day of their lives. At the same time, though, it is a description that can be applied to a hugely diverse range of individuals from chaotic, self-hating young men such as Danny to high-functioning manipulators like Tony or remorseless killers like Angela. Intelligent and dedicated men such as James Fallon seem to share their brain structure with criminal psychopaths, but to no more ill effect than a bit of social gruffness. How useful a concept is it that tries to lump all of these individuals together, and how concerning that in some parts of the world such an elastic concept can determine whether you live or die?

The reasons that someone commits a serious crime are unique, complex and difficult to unearth. That's why the best crime thrillers are almost always like archaeologies of the perpetrator's mind, peeling back layers of experiences and emotion that only make sense in relation to each other. This is what makes a psychopath, truly: not a diagnosis made by a test.

Notes

Preface

1. Although the Barlinnie Special Unit in Glasgow (Cooke, 1989) and HMP Grendon (Shuker and Sullivan, 2010) are isolated examples of success in rehabilitating very violent criminals with a likely diagnosis of psychopathy.

Introduction

1. I am going to use the term 'psychopath' in this book over the fairer description 'people with a diagnosis of psychopathic disorder' simply for reasons of brevity and the reader's patience. I apologise to anyone who is offended by this, but I hope the reader will also see that I understand there is an important distinction.
2. In fact this accusation is also applied, unfortunately, to a lot of people with a diagnosis of personality disorder: see NIHME, 2003, or Centre for Mental Health, 2018.
3. Rice and Harris, 1997.

Chapter One: The Masks of Psychopathy

1. Hare, 1991.
2. Ronson, 2011.
3. Huchzermeier, et al., 2008.

4. Viding, et al., 2005.
5. Blonigen, et al., 2006.
6. Cleckley, 1941.
7. Hare, 1980.
8. Ratiu, et al., 2004.
9. Macmillan, 2000.
10. Gale, et al., 2018.
11. Campbell-Meiklejohn, et al., 2012.
12. Blair, 2007.
13. Igoumenou, et al., 2017.
14. Fallon, 2013.
15. I use this word in the specific sense of John Bowlby's attachment theory (Bowlby, 1969), which is increasingly popular knowledge, especially among parents, but has its own relevance to psychopathy (e.g. Bowlby, 1946).
16. Nelson, 1994.
17. Rule, 1980.
18. Greenacre, 1945.
19. Frick and White, 2008.
20. Logan, 2011.
21. Forouzan and Cooke, 2005.
22. Quinsey, 2002.
23. Klein Tuente, et al., 2014.
24. Myers, etal., 2005.
25. Douglas, et al., 2006, Camp, Schmitt, et al., 2013.
26. Coid, et al., 2012.
27. Harris and Rice, 2006.

Chapter Two: Paul, The Hitman

1. Coid, et al., 2009.
2. Jackson, Craig, 'Nurse suspended over claims of inappropriate relationships with patients at secure Scots hospital,' *The Scottish Sun*, 19 October 2019,

https://www.thescottishsun.co.uk/news/4856692/
rowanbank-clinic-glasgow-nurse-nhs/.

Chapter Three: Tony, The Conman

1. For more on this sub-type see Heaver, 1944.
2. Office for National Statistics, 2018.

Chapter Four: Jason, The Liar

1. Cuellar, et al., 2007.
2. Mental Health Act (UK), 1983.
3. Li, et al., 2011.
4. Shao and Lee, 2017.
5. Garrett, et al., 2016.

Chapter Five: Arthur, The Parasite

1. Jolly, Jasper, 'Breaking Out: A man's redemption through rowing,' *Row 360*, 29 January 2016.
2. MacAvoy and Turley, 2016.

Chapter Six: Danny, The Borderline

1. This idea was first suggested by Anna Freud (1936).
2. Coid, et al., 2006.

Chapter Seven: Angela, The Remorseless

1. The Blom-Cooper inquiry into high-security mental health care of 1992 (see Blom-Cooper, et al., 1992) strongly criticised the 'prison-like' culture of the high-security hospitals at the expense of therapeutic input, and the influence of the Prison Officers' Association (POA) union on the delivery of nursing care. The traditional white uniforms were abolished and staff after that wore casual clothes.

2. A belief that may have had some merit as the sheriff's office was under investigation for racism, see Markon and McCrummen, 2010.
3. Knight, et al., 2017.
4. Maverty, 2014.
5. Boyd, 1993.
6. Arrigo and Griffin, 2004.
7. Strand and Belfrage, 2005.
8. For discussions of the way that psychopaths learn differently see Blair, et al., 2004, or Ling and Raine, 2018.

Chapter Eight: Eddie, The Redeemed

1. Felitti, et al., 1998.
2. Lerman and Iwata, 1995.
3. 'Extinction' is a Pavlovian concept that refers to the dying out of a particular conditioned reaction (such as Pavlov's dog salivating when it hears the bell, expecting food) – if the reward is not present for long enough, the reaction will eventually become extinct. See VanElzakker, et al., 2014.
4. Prochaska and DiClemente, 1992.

Chapter Nine: Psychopathy is Bad for your Health

1. Babiak and Hare, 2006.
2. Crick and Grotpeter, 1995.
3. Ishikawa, et al., 2001.
4. Gao and Raine, 2010.
5. Freestone, et al., 2020.
6. Brinkley, et al., 2001.
7. Viding, et al., 2005.

8. For a good history of the Henderson and its clinical model, see Manning, 1989.
9. Perry and Szalavitz, 2017.
10. Sutton, 2012.
11. Rosenbaum and Garfield, 1996.
12. Johnides, et al., 2017.
13. Perry, 2006.

Bibliography

Arrigo, B. A. and Griffin, A. (2004). Serial murder and the case of Aileen Wuornos: attachment theory, psychopathy, and predatory aggression. *Behav Sci Law*, 22(3): 375–393.

Babiak, P. and Hare, R. D. (2006). *Snakes in Suits: When Psychopaths Go to Work*. New York: Regan.

Bateman, A. and Fonagy, P. (2010). *Mentalization-based Treatment for Borderline Personality Disorders*. Oxford: Oxford University Press.

Blair, J. (2007). Dysfunctions of medial and lateral orbitofrontal cortex in psychopathy. *Ann N Y Acad Sci*, 1121: 461–479.

Blair, J., Mitchell, D. and Blair, K. (2005). *The Psychopath: Emotion and the Brain*. London: Wiley-Blackwell.

Blair, J., et al., (2004).

Passive avoidance learning in individuals with psychopathy: modulation by reward but not by punishment. *Personality and Individual Differences,* 37: 1179–1192.

Blom-Cooper, L., Brown, M., Dolan, R. and Murphy, E. (1992). *Report of the Committee of Inquiry into Complaints About Ashworth Hospital,* Cmnd 2028, vols 1 and 2. London: HMSO.

Blonigen, D. M., et al. (2006). Continuity and change in psychopathic traits as measured via normal-range personality: A longitudinal-biometric study. *J Abnorm Psychol,* 115(1): 85–95.

Boyd, C. J. (1993). The antecedents of women's crack cocaine abuse: Family substance abuse, sexual abuse, depression and illicit drug use. *J of Subst Abuse Treat,* 10(5): 433–438.

Bowlby, J. (1969). *Attachment and Loss, Vol. 1: Attachment* (2nd edn). New York: Basic Books.

Bowlby, J. (1946). *Forty-four Juvenile Thieves: Their Characters and Home-life* (2nd edn). London: Baillière, Tindall and Cox.

Brinkley, C. A., Schmitt, W. A., Smith, S. S. and Newman, J. P. (2001). Construct validation of a self-report psychopathy scale: Does Levenson's self-report psychopathy scale measure the same constructs as Hare's psychopathy checklist-revised? *Pers*, 31(7): 1021–1038.

Camp, J. P., et al. (2013). Psychopathic predators? Getting specific about the relation between psychopathy and violence. *J Consult Clin Psychol*, 81(3): 467–480.

Campbell-Meiklejohn, D. K., et al. (2012). Structure of orbitofrontal cortex predicts social influence. *Current Biology*, 22: 123–124.

Centre for Mental Health, Royal College of Nursing, British Association of Social Workers, Royal College of General Practitioners, The British Psychological Society, Anna Freud National Centre for Children and Families, MIND and Barnet, Enfield and Haringey NHS Trust (2018). *"Shining light in the dark corners of people's lives": The consensus statement for people with complex mental health difficulties who are diagnosed with a personality disorder.* London: MIND.

Cleckley, H. M. (1941). *The Mask of Sanity*. St Louis: C. V. Mosby.

Coid, J., et al. (2006). Prevalence and correlates of personality disorder in Great Britain. *Br J Psychiatry*, 188(5): 423–431.

Coid, J., et al. (2009). Psychopathy among prisoners in England and Wales. *International Journal of Law and Psychiatry*, 32(3): 134–141

Coid, J. and Yang, M. (2008). The distribution of psychopathy among a household population: categorical or dimensional? *Soc Psychiatry Psychiatr Epidemiol*, 43(10): 773–781.

Coid, J., Freestone, M. and Ullrich, S. (2012). Subtypes of psychopathy in the British household population: Findings from the national household survey of psychiatric morbidity. *Soc Psychiatry Psychiatr Epidemiol*, 47(6): 879–91.

Cooke, (1989). Containing Violent Prisoners: An Analysis of the Barlinnie Special Unit. *The British Journal of Criminology*, 29(2): 129–143.

Crick, N. R. and Grotpeter, J. K. (1995). Relational aggression, gender, and social-psychological adjustment. *Child Dev*, 66(3): 710–722.

Cuellar, A. E., Snowden, L. M. and Ewing, T. (2007). Criminal records of persons served in the public mental health system. *Psychiatr Serv*, 58(1): 114–120.

Douglas, K. S., Vincent, G. M. and Edens, J. F. (2006). Risk for criminal recidivism: The role of psychopathy. In Patrick, C. J. (ed.), *Handbook of Psychopathy*. Guilford: The Guilford Press, 533–554.

Fallon, J. (2013). *The Psychopath Inside: A Neuroscientist's Personal Journey Into the Dark Side of the Brain*. London: Penguin.

Felitti, Vincent J., et al. (1998) Relationship of childhood abuse and household dysfunction to many of the leading causes of death in adults. *Am J Prev Med*, 14(4): 245–258.

Forouzan, E. and Cooke, D. J. (2005). Figuring out la femme fatale: Conceptual and assessment issues concerning psychopathy in females. *Behav Sci Law*, 23(6): 765–778.

Freestone, M., Osman, M. and Ibrahim, Y. (in press, 2020). On the uses and abuses of narcissism for public health. *Br J Psychiatry*.

Freud, A. (1936) *The Ego and Mechanisms of Defence.* London: Routledge.

Frick, P. J. and White, S. F. (2008). Research review: The importance of callous-unemotional traits for developmental models of aggressive and anti-social behaviour. *J Child Psychol Psychiatry*, 49(4): 359–375

Gale, C., et al. (2018). Neonatal brain injuries in England: Population-based incidence derived from routinely recorded clinical data held in the National Neonatal Research Database. *Arch Dis Child Fetal Neonatal Ed*, 103(4): F301–F306.

Gao, Y. and Raine, A. (2010). Successful and unsuccessful psychopaths: A neurobiological model. *Behav Sci Law*. 28(2): 194–210.

Garrett, N., et al. (2016). The brain adapts to dishonesty. *Nat Neurosci*, 19: 1727–1732.

Greenacre, P. (1945). Conscience in the psychopath. *Am J Orthopsychiat*, 15(3): 495–509.

Hare, R. D. (1980). A research scale for the assessment of psychopathy in criminal populations. *Personality and Individual Differences*, 1(2): 111–119.

Hare, R. D. (1998). The Hare PCL-R: Some issues concerning its use and misuse. *Leg Criminol Psychol*, 3(Pt 1): 99–119.

Hare, R. D. (1991). *The Psychopathy Checklist: Revised*. Toronto: Multi-Health Systems.

Harris, G. T. and Rice, M. E. (2006). Treatment of psychopathy: A review of empirical findings. In Patrick, C. J. (ed.), *Handbook of Psychopathy*. Guilford: The Guilford Press, 555–572.

Heaver, W. L. (1944). A study of forty male psychopathic personalities before, during and after hospitalization. *Amer J Psychiat*, 100(3): 342–346.

Huchzermeier C., et al. (2008). Are there age-related effects in antisocial personality disorders and psychopathy? *J of Forensic Leg Med*, 15(4): 213–8.

Igoumenou, A., et al. (2017). Faces and facets: The variability of emotion recognition in psychopathy reflects its affective and antisocial features. *J Abnorm Psychol*, 126(8): 1066–1076.

Ishikawa, S. S., et al. (2001). Autonomic stress reactivity and executive functions in successful and unsuccessful criminal psychopaths from the community. *J Abnorm Psychol*, 110(3): 423–432.

Johnides, B. D., Borduin, C. M., Wagner, D. V. and Dopp, A. R. (2017). Effects of multisystemic therapy on caregivers of serious juvenile offenders: A 20-year follow-up to a randomized clinical trial. *J Consult Clin Psychol*, 85(4): 323–334.

Klein Tuente, S., de Vogel, V. and Stam, J. (2014). Exploring the criminal behavior of women with psychopathy: Results from a multicenter study into psychopathy and violent offending in female forensic psychiatric patients. *Int J Forensic Ment Health*, 13(4): 311–322.

Knight, B., Coid, J. W. and Ullrich, S. (2017). Non-suicidal self-injury in UK prisoners. *Int J Forensic Ment Health*, 16(2): 172–182.

Lerman, D. C. and Iwata, B. A. (1995). Prevalence of the extinction burst and its attenuation during treatment. *J Appl Behav Anal*, 28(1): 93–94.

Levin, J. and Wiest, J. B. (2018). *The Allure of Premeditated Murder: Why Some People Plan to Kill*. Lanham, MD: Rowman and Littlefield.

Li, A. S., Kelley, E. A., Evans, A. D. and Lee, K. (2011). Exploring the ability to deceive in children with autism spectrum disorders. *J Autism Dev Disord*, 41(2): 185–195.

Ling, S. & Raine, A. (2018). The neuroscience of psychopathy and forensic implications, *Psychology, Crime & Law,* 24:3: 296–312.

Logan, C. (2011). La femme fatale: The female psychopath in fiction and clinical practice. *MHRJ*, 16(3): 118–127.

MacAvoy, J. and Turley, M. (2016). *Redemption: From Iron Bars to Ironman*. Worthing: Pitch Perfect.

Macmillan, M. (2000). *An Odd Kind of Fame: Stories of Phineas Gage*. Boston: MIT Press.

Manning, N. (1989). *The Therapeutic Community Movement: Charisma and Routinisation*. London: Routledge.

Markon, J., McCrummen, S. (2010) Judge blocks some sections of Arizona Law. Washington: *The Washington Post*.

Maverty, J. (director). (2014). *Deadly Women: Heartless*, season 7, episode 9. Sydney, Australia: Beyond International.

Meloy, J. R. (2001). *The Mark of Cain: Psychoanalytic Insight and the Psychopath* (Kindle edn). London: Routledge.

Mental Health Act (UK) (1983). Section 1. Retrieved from http://www.legislation.gov.uk/ukpga/1983/20/contents.

Myers, W. C., Gooch, E. and Meloy, J. R. (2005). The role of psychopathy and sexuality in a female serial killer. *J Forensic Sci*, 50(3): 652–657.

Nelson, P. (1994). *Defending the Devil: My story as Ted Bundy's Last Lawyer*. New York: William Morrow.

National Institute for Mental Health in England (NIHME), (2003). *Personality Disorder: No Longer a Diagnosis of Exclusion*. London: Department of Health.

Office for National Statistics, UK (2018). *Sexual offending: Victimisation and the path through the criminal justice system*. London: Office for National Statistics.

Perry, B. D. (2006). Applying principles of neurodevelopment to clinical work with maltreated and traumatized children: The neurosequential model of therapeutics. In Webb, N. B. (ed.), *Social Work Practice with Children and Families: Working with traumatized youth in child welfare*. Guilford: Guilford Press, 27–52.

Perry, B. D. and Szalavitz, M. (2017). *The Boy Who Was Raised as a Dog, and Other Stories from a Child Psychiatrist's Notebook* (3rd edn). London: Basic Books.

Prochaska, J. O. and DiClemente, C. C. (1992). Stages of change in the modification of problem behaviors. *Prog Behav Modif*, 28: 183–218.

Quinsey, V. L. (2002). Evolutionary theory and criminal behavior. *Leg Criminol Psychol*, 7(1): 1–13.

Ratiu, P., et al. (2004). The tale of Phineas Gage, digitally remastered. *J Neurotrauma*, 21(5): 637–43.

Rice, M. E. and Harris, G. T. (1997). Cross-validation and extension of the violent risk-appraisal guide for child molesters and rapists. *Law and Hum Behav*, 21(2): 231–38.

Ronson, J. (2011). *The Psychopath Test*. London: Picador.

Rosenbaum, B. and Garfield, D. (1996), Containers, mental space and psychodynamics. Br *J Med Psychol*, 69(Pt 4): 281–297.

Rule, A. (1980). *The Stranger Beside Me: The Shocking Inside Story of Serial Killer Ted Bundy*. London: Sphere.

Shao, R. and Lee, T. M. C. (2017). Are individuals with higher psychopathic traits better learners at lying? Behavioural and neural evidence. *Transl Psychiatry*, 7(7): e1175.

Shuker, R. and Sullivan, E. (2010). *Grendon and the Emergence of Forensic Therapeutic Communities*. London: John Wiley & Sons, Ltd.

Strand, S. and Belfrage, H. (2005). Gender differences in psychopathy in a Swedish offender sample. *Behav Sci Law*. 23(6): 837–850.

Sutton, J. (2012). 'Patients with the disorder deserve to be helped'. *The Psychologist*. 25: 212–213.

VanElzakker, M. B., et al. (2014). From Pavlov to PTSD: The extinction of conditioned fear in rodents, humans, and anxiety disorders. *Neurobiol Learn Mem*, 113: 3–18.

Viding, E., Blair, R. J., Moffitt, T. E. and Plomin, R. (2005). Evidence for substantial genetic risk for psychopathy in 7-year-olds. *J Child Psychol Psychiatry*, 46(6): 592–597.

Acknowledgements

This book is really a product of a few of my more interesting interactions with people over the years and I am extremely grateful for all of them.

First of all, I am greatly indebted to my editor, Emma Smith at Ebury, who showed so much curiosity about the work behind *Killing Eve* and an oddly unshakeable faith in me despite my repeated deadline panics, ignorance of how to write popular science books and constant need to apologise for everything. In writing. Her comments and guidance improved this book considerably. I should also thank Charlotte Cole, the copyeditor, for making sense of large sections of the book that seemed, in hindsight, like nonsense.

Helen Czerski is a far better friend to me than I am to her, although she is pretty incredible at it so I don't feel at all bad acknowledging her superiority. She both inspired and motivated me throughout this process, including introducing me to Will Francis at Janklow and Nesbit, who has been an irreplaceable source of encouragement, pragmatism and behind-the-scenes negotiation that helped this book to happen.

Early in the writing process my great friend Jessica Gregson gave me the best possible advice anyone could receive in writing a book, which boiled down to 'just fucking write it, then worry about it', and which was exactly what I needed at the time when I only had 8,000 words written and a deadline barely months away. Hannah Jones, Georgina Mathlin and Landon Kuester at Queen Mary showed a quiet, encouraging interest in the book from the early days of me drunkenly unveiling it (under the working title of 'Killing Steve') and I hope this doesn't disappoint them.

A whole host of other people contributed to this book in various ways: firstly the man known only as Eddie on these pages was not just a subject of the chapter he starred in but an inspiration both in terms of his story and in his generosity of spirit and sense of humour. Lara Griffiths very generously gave her time to nudge me in some directions on some stories, and Dr Celia Taylor was greatly supportive of me, as she has been in the 11 years we have now worked together.

Cleo Van Velsen influenced my thinking about psychopathy and personality disorder more than anyone else and she is very present in these pages as an intellectual voice and a source of thought and compassion for those everyone else rejects. Jeremy Coid also influenced my thinking in complex ways, although sometimes I'm not sure whether he believes in psychopaths at all.

All the *Killing Eve* team at Sid Gentle treated me with great warmth and respect, which I hope I earned, but especially thank you Henrietta Colvin, Phoebe Waller-Bridge, Emerald Fennell, Elinor Day, Lee Morris, Chrissie Broadway and Sally Woodward Gentle. Vicky Jones is secretly responsible for the whole thing anyway, so she should probably go at the top of this section. Dan Crinnion – a formerly unsung but now Emmy-nominated editor – gave me shelter and firm, dad-based conversation at cast parties. Adeel Akhtar was terrific to work with on the Martin character, although people now think Martin's based on me. What's that about?

I would also like to thank Amandeep Singh at Ebury, Luna Centifanti, Alice Vincent, Rebecca Nicholson, Sophia Milsom, Claire Jones (née Moore), Sarah Linton, Nicola & Victoria Larder, and Rob Williams for helpful conversations that provoked me to think deeper about this work.

My wife, Lotte, has shown fathomless patience and understanding for this project as well as tirelessly and brilliantly parenting two young children often without my (admittedly inept) assistance on evenings and weekends. I love her greatly and without her this book would not have been a possibility.

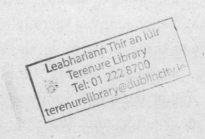

About the Author

Mark Freestone is a Senior Lecturer in the Centre for Psychiatry, Queen Mary University of London. He originally trained as a sociologist and has worked in prisons and forensic mental health services for over 15 years as a researcher and clinician, including in Category A prisons that house some of the UK's most notorious and high-risk criminals. He has also worked at high-security special hospitals as part of the Dangerous and Severe Personality Disorder (DSPD) Programme, which piloted new interventions for men and women in the UK with a diagnosis of psychopathy or a severe personality disorder. He was a consultant to series 1 and 2 of BBC America's *Killing Eve* and is an editor of the *Journal of Forensic Psychiatry and Psychology* and currently an advisor to NHS England on services for men and women with a diagnosis of severe personality disorder. He has published several academic articles on personality disorder, psychopathy and violence risk, but this is his first book.